MW01384675

THE MYSTERY OF PALMISTRY

P. Khurrana has pursued the subjects of astrology, mantras, numerology, sun signs, vaastu and tarot with great passion. Columnist, author and a devotee of Lord Shiva, he has featured as an astrologer on television channels such as *LIVE* INDIA, Zee (Punjabi), ETC (Punjabi) and on BIG FM (92.7). He is often invited for the mahurat of Bollywood films and is advisor to many actors and business tycoons.

To know more about the author, log on to www.astroindia. com.

Other Books by P. Khurrana

THE MYSTERY OF PALMISTRY

A Guide to the Art and Science of Palm Reading

P. KHURRANA

RUPA

First published in 2012 by
Rupa Publications India Pvt. Ltd.
7/16, Ansari Road, Daryaganj
New Delhi 110002

Sales Centres:

Allahabad Bengaluru Chennai
Hyderabad Jaipur Kathmandu
Kolkata Mumbai

ISBN: 978-81-291-1986-5

Second impression 2022

10 9 8 7 6 5 4 3 2

P. Khurrana asserts the moral right to be identified
as the author of this work.

Printed in India

Dedicated to

my mother, late Smt Raj Khurrana

Those who know astrology only indicate
what will take place in the future.
Who else except the creator Brahma
can say with certainty what will definitely happen?

Contents

Preface

Palmistry, the art and science of self-discovery, has been a part of our lives for ages. As we change and evolve with age, so do the lines on our hands.

Man has been studying the importance of these lines since the very existence of mankind. Even in ancient times, thumbprints were used for various purposes. Julius Caesar judged his men with the help of palmistry. By studying both hands—the non-dominant hand (past) and the dominant hand (present)—we can recognise the traceable link between our past behavioural patterns and our present personality, thoughts and experiences. With this understanding, we can shape our future in a constructive, fulfilling way, making positive choices regarding our work, our dealings with people around us and many other important aspects of life.

The practice of chiromancy is found all over the world, with numerous cultural variations. Those who practise it are generally called palmists, palm readers, hand readers, hand analysts or chirologists.

Chiromancy is generally regarded as a pseudoscience. The information outlined below is briefly representative of modern palmistry; there are many—often conflicting—interpretations of various lines and palm features across various 'schools' of palmistry.

Palmistry is also the term in older literature for sleight of hand.

The easiest way to verify it for oneself is by going to a palmist who knows nothing about you. If he is able to mention a few things that happened in the past and relate them to the present, then you will be far more receptive to what he says about the future. In the past, many distinguished philosophers wrote about and approved of this science, which led us to believe in its authenticity. But, at the same time, palmistry is an ancient art, and one that has many systems of interpretation. It is also an intuitive art that can be learned easily, by understanding a few basic things about the symbolism that is represented by the lines that run across the palm, the mounts (or fleshy parts) of the palm and the structure of fingers. In palmistry, the hand as a whole is divided into three different sections. The fingers represent the mind and the higher self. The middle of the palm represents day-to-day life and the conscious mind. The lower half of the palm represents primal instincts, health and basic drives of the subconscious. Palmistry is all about proportion, symmetry and distortions of what would be considered a perfectly formed hand.

Palmistry begins with the obvious and proceeds, by innumerable intricate steps of judgment and interpretation, to extreme details of the palm. Conclusions drawn from a palm reading can provide you with answers to questions you have regarding your life.

1

Introduction

Palmistry begins with the obvious and proceeds, by innumerable intricate steps of judgment and interpretation, to minute details of the palm. Conclusions from a palmistry reading can provide you with answers to questions regarding your life.

A palmist can interpret aspects of a person's life by reading the lines of the palm. An efficient palmistry practitioner will begin by examining both hands. In the case of a right-handed subject, the left hand is considered the 'birth hand', which shows inherited predispositions of character, while the right hand is thought to reflect individuality, flexibility and potential. For a left-handed subject, the opposite holds true.

It is the purpose of palmistry to teach you how to conquer the ancient art of divination by means of stated rules and not by intuition. The rules work accurately under all circumstances, whereas intuition comes and goes at its own sweet will, under the influence of some momentary excitement, a state of true clairvoyance, never to be fully relied upon. Palmistry is a well-established science, which attracts everyone. However, like every science, one needs patience to learn its deep intricacies and get its correct and true meaning. Every hand is a map of a life and every part of the hand, from the fingertips to the wrist, contains important markers to the points on the map. The roads and signposts in our hands are created by our nervous system. Our palms, fingers and hand postures tell a story about who we are and where we are going in our lives.

Each of our fingers and mounds has an astrological correspondence. Did you know that the size of your Saturn finger can say a lot about how you handle responsibilities? And that you can judge whether someone is being honest just by looking at the areas of the hand ruled by Mercury? By charting the astrological correspondences found in the palm, and understanding the mythologies of the gods and planets associated with each part of that map, it is possible to understand yourself and others by making simple observations about thumb size, finger length, gestures, lines and skin colour. It is important to look at both hands during a reading. Depending on which hand is active (usually seen as the hand you write with), in combination with the inactive hand, it shows where you have been in the past (passive), and where you are likely headed (active) in this life. Palmistry and hand analysis have intrigued humans throughout history. Nearly everyone enjoys a free hand reading. Perhaps the earliest interest in hand reading arose when the cave dwellers left their hand prints on cave walls over twelve thousand years ago. Throughout history, since writing was invented, thousands of documents have been created detailing palmistry and hand analysis techniques.

The palm is like a mirror that reflects the mind of a person from birth to death. Hands are servants of the body system, therefore, all that affects the system, affects them as well. A huge difference exists between the hands of different people with different temperaments. Almost everyone associated with medicine admits that different formations of nails indicate different diseases, and it is possible, from the nail alone, to predict whether a person is suffering from some disease.

There is a saying that the hand can express almost as much by its gestures and positions as the lips can by speech. Actually the hand by its direct communication with every portion of the brain, tells not only of the qualities active, but those dormant and those that will be developed as well. Palm reading or analysis is similar to reading body language. Our emotional energy affects every activity of our body. That energy is distributed at different levels throughout the body, more so in the hands. Palm analysts can analyse the different energies in the hands to identify how a person is functioning subconsciously in his life.

It is interesting to know that no two hands can be found to be alike even if they belong to twins. Another interesting fact is that certain peculiarities run in families for generations, and each succeeding race shows whatever that peculiar characteristic is in its temperament. Palm analysis helps us understand ourselves as well as others. It can help us identify many personal traits of strength, weakness, preference and character. The key to palm analysis is understanding how and which energies are displayed in the hands. One's hand is more like a photograph of that person.

2

Seven Basic Ethics of Palm Reading

1. Give adequate time while learning and do not be hasty.
2. Be honest with yourself about your knowledge.
3. Do not guess. Stay silent if not sure.
4. Give each part and section a thorough reading.
5. The palmist should sit at a convenient distance from the client so that the hand is clearly visible and the client does not feel uncomfortable.
6. The palmist and client should face each other and not sit side by side as it may be an uneasy setting.
7. The palmist should not move the hand repeatedly in order to read it.

WHAT IS THE AUSPICIOUS TIME TO READ THE HAND?

Generally, it is believed that early morning is the best time for reading since the blood flow is stronger during the morning. It is also believed that it is better for a reading if the client has not eaten after waking up. However, I am of the opinion that a few hours after waking up is the best time for a reading, since by then, the colour of the hand is more prominent and therefore easier to read and understand. If the palmist is unsure of a specific part of the hand and finds that the lines are unclear, then the best thing to do is to press the hand on that specific part and release the pressure, so that when the blood flows again in that area, the lines are seen easily. This provides the palmist with more clarity sans any doubt.

USEFUL TIPS

1. One should be judicious while speaking each word to the client.
2. One should be clear in his speech and meaning so that there is no room for misunderstanding.
3. One should avoid excessive detailing without being asked to do so.
4. One should always remember to be humble.
5. One should avoid giving direct answers as far as possible.
6. If one wants to pursue palmistry as a profession, then it is vital to take guidance from an experienced palmist and to regard him as your teacher.
7. One should not read the palm under the influence of intoxicants.
8. One should not read at a social gathering.

POINTS TO REMEMBER

Be Objective

It is always better to say something general when telling someone's future. Being specific may create a problem for the palmist as well as the client. Specifying the exactness of an event may be problematic, especially if the palmist is in doubt. Or else, it can raise questions on his credibility.

Positive Attitude

Encouraging words should be said to a client who is under stress or anxiety. Rather than focusing on the negative aspects of one's life, it is advised to focus on the positive aspects. This is done to relieve him of the tension and direct him towards positivity. It may also help him rise above his problems.

Study

Palmistry is a study and the accuracy of the readings and predictions is difficult to determine. Predictions can be considered hints towards what is to happen in a person's life rather than something that is bound to happen. They can be termed as facilitators which help determine the events that may take place in a person's life so that preventive or corrective measures can be taken. One must always remember that there is nothing as uncertain as one's life.

Tactful

The lines and markings on a person's hand keep changing; therefore, one must not guess when one is not sure or when one is not able to read clearly. It is better not to have an opinion or comment when one is uncertain.

Physical Condition

The first and foremost thing to look at is the client's lifeline. If it is positive, it determines the events and prospects in a person's life. Therefore, lifeline should be prioritised. The next line to be studied is the person's head line which provides knowledge about the various vital decisions in the client's life.

A person's nails provide us knowledge about his health. If the colour of the nails is pale then it is a reflection of unstable health and if the colour of the nails is pinkish, it reflects sound health. If factors indicate negative health, then the client can be informed so that he can take more care of himself. It can be termed as a warning for the client.

3

Methods of Reading

SHORT READING

It refers to the general understanding of all the lines that are present in a hand. Though it is a narrow form of reading, it is likely to be true with respect to its meaning. It is an essential and vital form of reading; it is precise and consumes less time. It mainly focuses on the basic and prominent lines of the hand and lacks detailing. It is a quick view at a person's past, present and future. The numerous other determinants in a person's hand which give insight into his life are not studied in this form of reading. If those other factors are included in the study, only then can a palmist provide a detailed analysis of the client's life.

AVERAGE READING

This form of reading, along with the study of various lines of the hand, includes the study of the nails and the shape of the hand. This provides additional information and a better understanding of the client's life. It further helps the palmist to arrive at a more definite conclusion regarding various aspects of the person's life. This form of reading evokes the personal instinct in the palmist and improves the accuracy of his reading. It provides more satisfaction to the client as well as the palmist as he is more confident and clear about his study.

COMPLETE READING

In this form of reading, the palmist is able to apply his personal skill along with the reading of the hand. The knowledge he gets from reading the client's hand is supplemented with his various observations and experience, giving his reading an edge and better results. This can only be done if the palmist has considerable experience.

THE RIGHT AND THE LEFT HAND

Each of the two hands has its own distinctive features which help us know the various other features and aspects of our life. Therefore, in order to understand the various unique and significant features associated with each hand, I will specify the difference in our hands from a palmist's point of view. The first and foremost thing to know is whether a person is left-handed or right-handed. Most of the people are right-handed which means that the right hand is their active hand. Their left hand signifies the character traits that the person was born with, and the right hand signifies the outcome of a person's life in accordance with the opportunities that came along his way. Earlier, the left hand was considered more significant due to its closeness to the heart as it is the most vital organ of the body. It was also believed that the left hand governs the emotional processes of a person.

At a later stage, the right hand was considered the main determinant of a person's life and his character, since it was considered the hand of labour which provides experience and livelihood. Due to its prominence, in practical terms, it was considered more significant.

Therefore, the most important thing to do is to determine whether a person is right-handed or left-handed as it is a vital factor while reading about a person's life and its various other features. A person's active hand has more strength than the inactive one. The active hand helps in knowing a person's present and how he shapes up in his future, whereas the inactive hand bestows knowledge about the person's past.

THE LEFT HAND

This hand gives insight into the traits that a person was born with, which may be an outcome of his past lives. It gives knowledge about the person that we are born as and denotes the flaws and qualities that we possessed when we were given the gift of life. The lines and markings of the hand keep changing. Many a times, the personality of an individual changes accordingly. This hand can be termed as the storehouse of knowledge regarding his persona.

THE RIGHT HAND

The right hand is a reflection of our present and future. This is actually where a palmist can determine the client's future. The left hand signifies the possibilities that may come up in a person's life in accordance with his capabilities, whereas the right hand signifies the way those possibilities have taken shape eventually. If there is an indication of the happening of an event in the left hand but not indicated in the right hand, it symbolizes that those possibilities may not have taken a successful road. It simply states that there was a possibility of the event taking place but the person may have missed an opportunity for it to materialize. Similarly, if certain events which are not indicated in the left hand are present in the right hand, it means that the person has opened the horizons of possibility and opportunity to create those events.

4

Various Shapes of the Hand

The shape of the hand of a person indicates a lot about the person's character and his traits. Every person is hand has a unique shape, and this shape reflects the nature and personality of that person. So, to understand these traits, we need a thorough understanding of the various shapes of hands. Therefore, after gaining knowledge of the same, we can identify the positive as well as the negative aspects of a person's character, and help the person in curbing the negative areas and enhancing his positive qualities. The various hand shapes provide valuable knowledge which a palmist can put to use while reading the various lines and markings so as to relate these with each other.

There are two types of basic hand shapes:

1. The Conic hand; it is considered a creative person's hand.
2. The Square hand; it is considered the hand of the humble.

The tips of the fingers play a vital role in knowing about a person's character. Sometimes, the shape of one hand varies from the other, though it does not happen very often.

THE CONIC HAND – IMAGINATIVE

A person who possesses the conic hand is artistic and imaginative. The tips of the fingers are round and the overall look of the hand is sleek while the palm is longer. Such people have a thirst to achieve more and keep working till they are satisfied with their efforts. They also have a need for change rather than stability. They are impatient by nature and may find their routine monotonous very often due to which they may constantly look for change. Because of their love for creativity, they will always be inclined to being an artist, a poet, a writer or an actor. They may also be their own critic and a little too harsh on themselves because they constantly want to achieve more. Rather than financial satisfaction in their work, they strive for personal satisfaction. They prioritise their personal achievements over monetary gain.

They are of a conflicting or indecisive nature. They find it hard to make up their minds regarding even the smallest of things. They are likely to be well-settled and appreciated professionally.

THE SQUARE HAND – HUMBLE

The overall shape of this type of hand is square. The palm is bigger than the fingers. The tips of the fingers are square in shape. The wrist is thick. People who possess square hands are realistic but conservative in nature.

They are organized and logical in their approach towards life. They prove to be successful professionally due to their eye for detail. They can be stubborn and will not be flexible in their beliefs and opinions. They are usually inexpressive in nature and tend to take ample time before establishing a connection at an emotional level with someone. Their commitment is of utmost importance due to which they prove to be very good friends. Business sector proves to be extremely beneficial for them. It can be exceedingly difficult to judge the way they feel as they rarely show their emotions.

THE PHILOSOPHIC HAND – SENSIBLE

This type of hand can be differentiated on the basis of the bony structure of the fingers. Because of this, the knuckles seem prominent. The fingers are long and sleek and the fingertips are slightly rounded in shape.

This type of hand signifies knowledge, intelligence and insight. Such people are unlikely to take any wrong decisions in life. They believe in leading life on the basis of principles and beliefs, and materialistic success does not attract them. They are likely to lead a simple but a spiritually-rich life. Their lives revolve around trying to be a better person resulting in their not being very successful professionally. These traits make them very caring and giving in relationships. They are inclined towards strong religious beliefs. They are likely to be extremely introspective in nature. Their level of tolerance is exceptionally high. They like their company and even in the company of many people they are likely to be alone. They tend to detest people who are materialistic in nature. Whatever profession they choose, they put deep thought and dedication into it.

THE PSYCHIC HAND – INSIGHTFUL

In this type of hand, the fingers are longer than the palm and the fingertips are thinner compared to the fingers. These types of hands are sleek and fragile to look at. They are also usually small in size.

The shape of these hands is considered the most beautiful of all, though they are rare to come across. It is termed as a psychic hand because this type of hand is pointed at the fingertips making it easy to receive positive vibrations and energy from the surroundings. This proves to be an intuitive instinct for the person which may not be possible for a person who has square fingertips. They are not worldly in nature and may prove professionally unsuccessful. They have an element of immaturity and innocence due to which they may need guidance frequently in their life. They lead a simple life and do not tend to understand the complications of life. They are easy to dupe and should be extra cautious in life and relationships. They are artistic and inventive in nature and possess a tendency to be submissive.

THE SPATULATE HAND

This type of hand can be distinguished from the other hands on the basis of the shape of the fingers. The fingertips are square, though thicker in shape than in a square hand. The spatulate hand is restless and quick. People with this type of hand believe in living their lives according to their rules and are extremely independent. They have freshness in their approach towards managing their personal and professional lives. They are also dominating. It is difficult for them to follow rules and limit their desires due to restrictions of logic and reason. They are likely to follow their heart. They may also have a not-so-ordinary attitude. They are fun-loving and tend to make friends very easily and hence they are likely to have an active social life. The inventive streak in their character makes them successful in fields relating to media, entertainment, architecture and theatre.

THE MIXED HAND

In this type of hand, the shape of the fingers is not specific; it is a mixture of various shapes. The shape of the fingers and the palm resembles various types of hand shapes—conic, square, philosophic, etc. This type of people have the ability to be flexible and adapt themselves to circumstances and situations. They are proficient in the art of speaking. Professionally, they prove to be extremely successful in banking and insurance sectors due to their verbal skills. They are fiercely independent as they are proud to be what they are; they are honest about their flaws and shortcomings. They are brave while facing any crisis and are extremely confident while dealing with competition.

THE BASIC HAND

This type of hand is small with short but broad fingers. People with laborious jobs usually have such hands. They are down-to-earth by nature and do not appreciate pomp and show. Having had to struggle during the initial stages of their life, they remain grounded in their values and principles even if they achieve fame and success. They do not have an active social life. They usually have a very close circle of friends. They are extremely hard-working professionally but success does not come easily to them. They have a tendency to be harsh in their words and are unlikely to be politically correct in their approach. If professionally successful, they prove to be a benchmark for others. They can be extremely difficult to cope with as employers since they follow principles religiously and may expect their employees to do the same. This type of hand is mostly possessed by farmers.

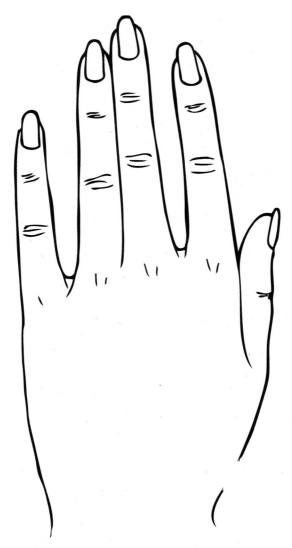

Psychic Hand

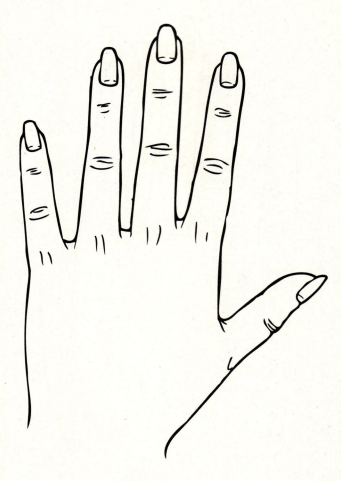

Conic Hand

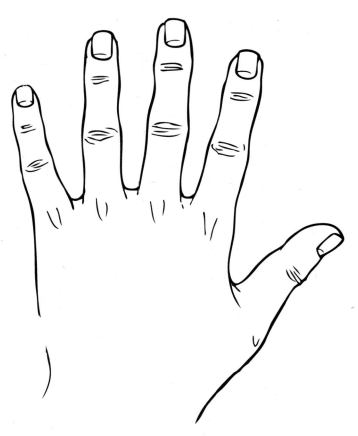

Philosophic Hand

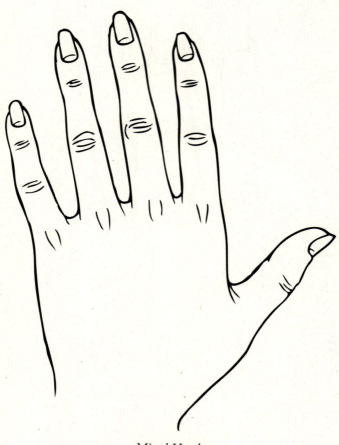

Mixed Hand

5

Size of the Hand and Personality

It is not just the shape of the hand that reflects the personality of a person but also the size of the hand that narrates the person's character. A large hand influences a person's personality more strongly than a person whose hand is small in size. Ironic as it may sound, people with large hands have an eye for detail and prefer doing delicate jobs or jobs that require excessive attention, whereas people with small hands are likely to take up big projects.

LARGE HANDS

People with large hands are more inclined towards jobs which require extra care and caution. They are also usually hard to please and have their standards set for everything. They find it hard to accept anything which does not meet their standards.

SMALL HANDS

People with small hands are likely to be creative and fun to be with, but have the tendency to be unorganized at times. They have a flexible attitude towards life and like to take life as it comes. Their goals and direction in life are extremely clear to them and they hardly ever deviate from it.

SKIN TEXTURE

If the texture of the skin is rough, it does not necessarily mean that it is due to hard work. The skin is coarse if the pores on the skin are prominent. Usually, it is more noticeable at the back of the hand. People with rough skin are usually more practical, tend to have a more carefree approach towards life and are humble. They are likely to be dominating in character. They are also straightforward.

A person with smooth skin is likely to be sensitive. Such a person has love for art and beauty, has refined tastes, is generally diplomatic and a good conversationalist. Such people are extremely conscious about the way they look, and likewise, the way others present themselves is of vital importance to them.

HAIR ON THE BACK OF THE HANDS

The hair on the back of the hand also signifies various characteristics of a person. It further helps us to know the personality of an individual. Earlier, palmists had a narrow and different approach towards this aspect of the hand. However, I believe, if studied carefully, it can be easily associated with a person's character.

The hair on the back of the hand also indicates physical and emotional strength of a person. Years ago, people considered a person with thick hair on the back of his hand to be emotionally unattached and vindictive in nature. Hair on our body grows from within us bringing out our character, personality traits and habits.

In other words, we can say that they speak a language of their own.

A person with light hair is likely to be sensitive and emotionally weak in relationships, whereas, a person with thick hair is likely to be ambitious and practical in his approach. People with thin and fine hair are creative and sophisticated in nature though they have a submissive attitude.

Fine and light hair

Such a person is ambitious and not worldly in his approach to life.

Thick hair

Such a person is dominating in nature and has a strong sense of direction in life.

No hair

Such a person is extremely organized and neat in nature.

Black hair

This type of person is loving and caring and keeps his relations close to his heart due to which he can be overly possessive and protective. But they have a tendency to be inexpressive.

Red hair

Such people are short-tempered and have mood swings.

Brown hair

People with brown hair are extremely humble and prove to be great friends since they value those around them.

Hair on the thumb

Such a person is extremely creative and broad-minded.

Hair on all the fingers

This indicates that a person is hard-working

Thick and rough hair

Such a person can be harsh from outside but is in fact a soft person by nature.

6

Significance of Various Fingers

Generally people associate palmistry with just the lines on the palm, not knowing the important role that the fingers play in determining the direction of a person's life. Each finger on our hand narrates a different story. It describes our personality in its own way. A finger's length, size, thickness and shape, all have different meanings to it. For example, a person with long fingers is likely to be patient and creative whereas a person with short fingers is inclined to take hasty decisions in life. The texture of the skin, the hair on our hands, and fingers also give us an insight into our life and traits. The shape and the texture of the nails help us know a person's basic nature. A person's character can be understood only by understanding the significance of different types of fingers.

THE FINGERS

The first finger (Index finger, Jupiter)
The second finger (Middle, Saturn)
The third finger (Ring, Apollo)
The fourth finger (Little, Mercury)

EFFECT OF ITS POSITIONING

The Jupiter Finger

Normally, the index finger is aligned above the other fingers at the base with the palm. But if it is aligned below the other fingers then the person is likely to suffer from lack of confidence and be submissive in nature. Such a person will have to face some struggle in life.

The Saturn Finger

Having a middle finger lower than the other fingers is very rare. In this case a person may have to face various hardships in life. Such a person is likely to be emotionally weak and will find it rather tough to face emotional setbacks in life.

The Apollo Finger

If a person's ring finger is placed below the rest of the fingers on the hand, then the person is likely to be extremely giving in nature. This type of persons will lack personal happiness due to this trait which might hurt them in return. This will make others take advantage of their innocence and immaturity.

The Mercury Finger

The little finger is usually placed lower than the rest of the fingers. But if this finger is placed at the same level as other fingers, then the person will be extremely successful in his professional life. Success and happiness will come easily to them without putting in much effort for it.

CLASSIFICATION OF VARIOUS FINGERS

The Jupiter Finger

This finger symbolizes dignity, control, leadership qualities and confidence. It determines the level of idealism and the philosophy of a person's life. It also reflects a person's level of ego. It tells us how faithful a person is in his relationships. This finger helps us know the level of authority and control in a person. The extent of these traits depends on the length of the index finger.

If the first and the third finger are approximately of the same length, the person will have a sensible and practical outlook towards life. Such a person will be ambitious in a balanced way; he will know the direction of his goals and will work towards them without overdoing it.

If the first finger is longer than the third finger, then the person will be overly ambitious due to which he may even tend to ignore his personal life and health. Such a person can be overly demanding and authoritative and he may not have a good equation with his colleagues and subordinates.

When the first finger is noticeably shorter than the third finger, then the person will be inclined towards taking wrong decisions in life as he makes these decisions in haste. But he is thoughtful and kind. This person will lack confidence due to which he will face professional difficulties. He will be easily intimidated in the presence of another person.

If the shape of the finger is straight then the person will be liberal, creative and reasonably ambitious in life. The person will have considerable confidence and will be efficient.

If the shape of the finger curves towards the second finger, he will lack confidence and will have the tendency to be selfish. Such a person will be dependent on the people around him for support.

The Saturn Finger

This finger symbolises awareness, honesty and cautiousness. This is the longest finger of the hand. The length of this finger helps us know whether the person will follow intuition or logic. It represents study, responsibility, reliability and watchfulness. It tells us if the person is very possessive and loving. This finger brings about consistency in the life of a person.

If this finger is smaller than the normal size, then the person will be reckless and carefree in nature. He will not be very dependable. This person does not like the company of people and prefers being by himself. Such a person also has a tendency to be boring and will therefore not have a big social circle. He will have very few friends and may be misunderstood many a time for being a quiet person. The middle finger balances the attitude of a person and a short finger makes the person negative in nature.

The length of this finger helps us to know how the person will function while making most of the decisions of his life, his emotions or his logic. A person whose Saturn finger is longer than the normal size is likely to be a loner and will detest being around a lot of people. Such a person also has a tendency to be pessimistic in nature. He will strive to achieve his goals but will have to work hard to achieve them. He can be dull company due to which he will have a very small circle of friends.

If this finger is close to the third finger, then it indicates that the person has an independent nature with an imaginative bent of mind. If this finger is close to the index finger, then the person will be overly ambitious and determined. He will be stubborn enough to achieve what he desires.

The Apollo Finger

This finger is related to one's contentment and happiness. It is also known as the ring finger. This finger relates to living on the spur of the moment. It also relates to the sensitive side of the individual's personality. This finger deals with the personal achievements of an individual. Mostly, this finger is almost always the same size as the index finger. Such people love having a big social circle and enjoy being the centre of attraction. They do not have a very futuristic approach and love to go with the flow. This can put them in tricky situations at certain times. But this nature can also prove to be a boon for them in certain professions like mass media and theatre. This finger also determines the level of imagination in a person. It relates to the person's love for beauty as well. Therefore, such people will have a tendency to be at their best at all times and will often be known for their sophisticated tastes. These people are flexible at all times and in all situations which will make them successful in trying times.

Normally, this finger's length touches the base of the nail of the Saturn finger or somewhere up to the middle part of the nail of the Saturn finger. If the length exceeds this, then the person will be fortunate in life. Such a person will also be confident and courageous in nature. They have a determined approach to life and will have the tendency to be hard-working when they decide on achieving something. Their spontaneous nature will at times make them take wrong decisions in life.

If this finger is smaller than the normal size, then the person will not be able to fully utilize all the opportunities that he comes across. Such a person is not able to realize his worth and put it to use. A person with a short Apollo finger will also be temperamental and may have a small social circle because of his mood swings.

Ideally, this finger should be straight in shape, which shows that the person is emotionally stable and balanced. This person will be creative and well-organized which leads to his being professionally successful. Slowly but steadily, he will be able to achieve his goals and fulfil his desires.

If the Apollo finger inclines towards the middle finger, then the person will follow his head instead of heart. Such a person will not follow his innovative instinct and rather choose a profession that does not appeal to his heart.

If the Apollo finger is inclined towards the little finger, then the person will choose a profession that is creative. This person will have contentment in his line of work. Such a person will not be able to fully utilize his potential as long as he is not doing what he wants to do.

The Mercury Finger

The Mercury finger, also known as the little finger, is named after Mercury, the Roman messenger of the gods. Therefore, it relates to the power of expression, amiability and psychological alertness in a person. It has the power effect and can be persuasive. It also relates to monetary and financial aspects of life along with physical desire in a person. This finger also provides an insight into the intensity of sex drive in a person.

This finger determines the intensity of communication skills possessed by a person. It also determines the degree of flexibility or how adaptable the person is. It makes a person highly focused and determined in his goals and objectives.

Normally, the length of this finger touches the very first joint of the Apollo finger or the ring finger. A person who possesses a mercury finger with an average length has the ability to stand up for what he believes in. He will not be dominating and will have the strength to face the consequences of his values and viewpoints. He will have a socialistic attitude and the tendency to try and change the unethical practices around him.

If this finger is long in size, then the person will possess not only good communication skills but also noteworthy writing skills. Such a person may prove to be a successful scriptwriter or author. Such persons generally make great poets as their writing skills are related to great levels of creativity and imagination. The communication skills of a person are directly related to the length of the finger. The longer the finger the better a person will be at self-expression. Such a person will be sexually active and adventurous. This type of person considers his sex life to be highly important.

A short Mercury finger implies that the person will not be expressive in nature. Such a person will have the tendency to keep his emotions bottled up inside. Therefore, such people have a very small social circle as they do not easily become friendly and comfortable with others. They will also tend to have a difficult nature and only their close ones can realise and discern what they feel. Such people will also have a dissatisfactory sex life.

A person whose Mercury finger is straight is transparent, trustworthy and honest in his dealings. If this finger is bent, then the person will not be fair in his dealings. A bent little finger also denotes a person who likes to communicate but is sometimes at a loss to put it into words.

The Thumb

The thumb is the most vital of all the fingers in a hand. It is considered as the leader of all the fingers in palmistry since it represents the mind, logic and determination. The thumb reveals almost all the aspects of an individual's personality. Therefore, palmists attach a lot of importance to the thumb. It signifies the energy, mental strength and assertiveness in a person.

The thumb signifies logic, and therefore affects our mind and psychology. It is believed that the thumb guides us towards the right direction in life. There are some palmists who read only the thumb.

The size of our thumb denotes the level of our confidence and communication related to self-expression. The size of our thumb greatly affects the outcome of our palm. The imperfections of our palm can be rectified or minimized by a large thumb and vice versa. The outcome of our life is greatly determined by the size of the thumb.

People who possess an average-sized thumb are fairly ambitious, family-oriented and have a tendency to not fully utilize their potential. An average thumb extends half way up to the bottom phalange of the index finger.

If the size of the thumb is smaller than normal, then the person will be temperamental. He will have the desire to achieve but will lack in efforts and driving spirit. He will also have the tendency to be indecisive at times and be inclined to take wrong decisions at times.

If the thumb is longer than the average size, then the person will be ambitious and hard-working. Such a person will make every possible effort to achieve his goals. Such people are also energetic and full of life due to which they will have the thirst to achieve more.

The positioning of the thumb also helps us determine the traits of a person. The thumb is set at a normal position when it is half-way between the wrist and the index finger. In this case, the person will be able to fully utilize his potential.

If the thumb is set at a level higher than average, which means it is closer to the index finger, then the person will be inflexible in nature and would be stubborn. Due to an incessant need to fulfil his desires, such a person will have the tendency to be selfish at times. He will also be extremely possessive about his close ones.

If the thumb is set at a lower level, which implies that it is closer to the wrist, then the person will have the propensity to be selfless and giving in nature. Such people are spontaneous and believe in going with the flow. They are fiercely independent and fun-loving.

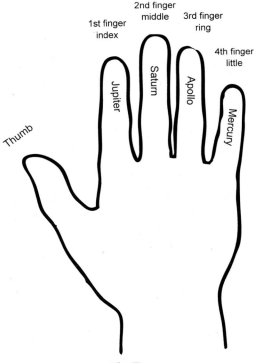

The Fingers

THE WIDTH OF THE FINGER

Thin Finger

This type of finger denotes a creative bent of mind. They are extremely organized and disciplined in nature. They love nature and work towards the well-being of the society. They are idealistic and loving.

Medium Finger

This type of finger makes a person stubborn and dominating. They have a tendency to be intimidated by artificial beauty, though they have a refined taste; they will be sophisticated in nature. They will tend to have mixed traits which may not be entirely negative or positive.

Thick Finger

A big or fat finger implies that the person will be extremely ambitious and worldly in character. This type will possess a soft heart but will seem to be a tough person. They can also be undemonstrative. They will have a love for luxury which leads constant striving to fulfil their needs and desires.

GAPS BETWEEN THE FINGERS

The gaps between a person's fingers further help us to know about an individual. If there is a prominent gap between the first and second finger, it signifies that the person is assertive and self-confident. Such a type of person religiously follows his beliefs and principles. Such a person is definite about his direction in life and strongly follows what he believes in.

A prominent gap between the second and the third finger denotes that the person is a spendthrift and is likely to make impulsive decisions in life. Such a person is not futuristic.

A noticeable gap between the third and the fourth finger is very common. This type of a person is fiercely independent and likes to live his life by his own rules. He will have a tendency to be inexpressive at times. But, such people also have an impressive personality since they are very good with words. They also have an eye for beauty.

If all the fingers of a person are widely spaced, then the person is friendly, social and cheerful in nature.

If all the fingers of a person are closely spaced, then the person is likely to be an introvert and extremely careful. This type of person may also be negative and possess a fault-finding attitude.

Therefore, those little spaces between the fingers, which we may not pay attention to, are actually much more than mere spaces. They can foretell a person's character and personality.

TEXTURE OF THE FINGER

Smooth Texture

If the texture of the skin of the fingers is fine, then the person will possess a high level of flexibility. He will be creative in nature but inclined towards quickness in actions and therefore hasty. He will tend to get stressed out very easily and be temperamental. He is emotionally active leading him to take decisions with the heart rather than with logic.

Coarse Texture

If the texture of the skin is rough, then the person is likely to have a strong logical mind, and will weigh the pros and cons of every situation before taking any decision. He can be stubborn and inflexible. Such people are extremely worldly and are not easy to deceive. They are usually practical and will rarely get emotionally attached. They value their personal life and will hardly ever gossip. They also have the tendency to become short-tempered when they have to deal with carelessness or lack of professionalism.

POSITIONING OF FINGERS

It refers to the placement of the fingers on the palm. This positioning of the fingers can also provide us an insight into the life of a person. It is determined according to the placement of the fingers at their base. They are usually of two types:

Straight-line Position

In this type of positioning, all the fingers are aligned in the form of a straight line at the base adjoining the palm. This type of positioning is rare and denotes prosperity and achievement in personal and professional life.

Arc-shaped Position

In this type of positioning, the fingers are placed in such a manner that the base of the fingers is in the form of an arc from the index fingers towards the little finger. This type of placement of fingers indicates a hard-working life and great efforts will be needed to fulfil goals.

7

In Relation to the Lines

The rules in relation to the lines are: they should be clear and well marked, neither broad nor pale in colour; they should also be free from all breaks, islands or irregularities of any kind.

1. Lines that are very pale indicate want of robust health and lack of energy and decision.
2. Lines red in colour indicate a sanguine, hopeful disposition; they show an active, robust temperament.
3. Yellow lines, indicative of biliousness and liver trouble, are indicators of a nature self-contained, reserved and proud.
4. Lines very dark in colour, almost black, tell of a melancholy, grave temperament and also indicate a haughty, distant nature, one usually very revengeful and unforgiving.
5. Lines may appear, diminish, or fade, which must always be borne in mind when reading the hand. The province of the palmist, therefore, is to warn the subject of approaching danger by pointing out the evil tendencies in his nature. It is purely a matter of the client's will whether he will try to overcome these tendencies, and it is by seeing how nature has modified

the tendencies in the past that the palmist can predict whether they will be overcome in the future. In reading the hand, no single evil mark must be accepted as decisive. If the evil is dominant, almost every principal line will show its effect, and both hands must be consulted before the final decision is announced. A single sign in itself only shows the tendency; when, however, other lines follow the sign, the danger is almost a certainty.

MOUNTS

There are nine mounts on a palm which are named after the nine planets. It symbolises the relation of palmistry with astrology. They are called mounts because they are raised masses of skin on the palm. These mounts influence the lines that pass through them or touch them. These mounts provide us with an insight into the various aspects of our life. The four mounts at the base of the four fingers have the same name as the fingers. The other five mounts are located on the outer part of the palm.

These mounts help us know which area of a person's life will play a dominant role in his future. They also inform us about the choice of career that a person is more likely to be successful in or will be drawn to. It is believed that numerous ends of various nerves are collected in these mounts which make them powerful and influential. It is not necessary for the mounts of one hand to be identical with the mounts of the other hand; they may differ.

The size of the mount also plays a vital role in determining its influence and importance. If a mount is bigger in size in comparison to the other mounts, then the subject which is indicated by that mount, will have a better scope in comparison to the other aspects of life. Similarly, a mount which is smaller in size indicates that the area which is symbolized by that mount will not be dominant. Ideally, the hand should have balanced mounts. Usually, the size of the mounts is the same and the difference is usually not very prominent.

A large mount possesses more power than a mount that is flat. Larger mounts indicate more dominance of that area in a person's life and more drive in those areas. Larger mounts are also the areas of our liking and interest to which we naturally pay more attention, and tend to put in more effort in that direction. This is also another reason why mounts play a leading role in a person's life. Subsequently, an individual is likely to achieve success in these areas.

The size of the mount tends to change with time. It also reflects the mental changes that keep occurring within us and our character. Mounts also change momentarily according to the mood swings of a person. This difference can be observed after a vigorous activity and after a good sleep.

The most prominent mount is the mount of Venus which is at the base of the thumb. This mount determines the sex drive in an individual. It reflects the quality of the sex life of a person. The size of this mount tends to change according to the state of sexual satisfaction of a person at that particular time. If some other mount appears to be more prominent than the mount of Venus, then the qualities and traits of that mount will dominate the character of a person.

The placement of mounts also reflects a lot of different characteristics in an individual. The top of the mount can aid us to know whether a mount is accurately placed on the palm. If the mount is placed directly under the middle of the base of the finger then it is said to be rightly placed. Such a person will have fulfilment in those areas which are dominated by that mount. But if the mount is more inclined towards the next finger, then the qualities of the adjoining finger will also influence the character of the mount and eventually the individual.

The size of the finger which adjoins the mount also plays a key role in determining the extent of the effect of a particular mount on an individual. The influence of the mount will be comparatively less if the finger is thin or small than if the finger is thick or big.

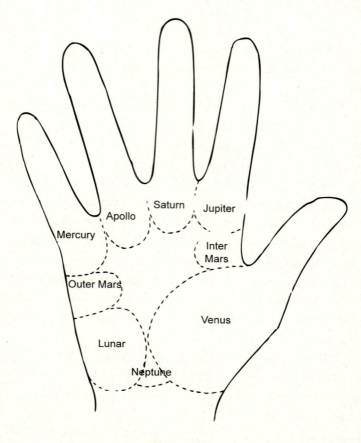

The Mounts

The Mount of Jupiter

The mount of Jupiter is located at the bottom of the index finger. If this mount is full in size, it shows that the person is dominating and likes to take charge of situations. This type of person is commanding and prefers things to be done his way. Such persons love their freedom and are fun loving. They are social and prove to be great company. They have an idealistic bent of mind and are rational in their approach towards life. They can be immensely stubborn when it comes to their beliefs and principles.

This type of persons are likely to be positive in their attitude towards life and will prove to be go-getters. They are immensely secure and self-assured which keeps their life radiant on personal and professional fronts. They prove to be good leaders because of their idealistic and fair approach. Though they may be an object of envy for many, they will be admired as leaders and as persons. They are caring and affectionate in personal relationships which keep them emotionally secure and content. They are very determined and once they set their mind on a goal they are unlikely to let it go until they achieve it. This attitude helps them climb the ladder of success.

They have a giving nature and are likely to be involved in charity and social work as well. The happiness of their close ones is extremely important to them. They may become political or religious leaders due to their tremendous public-speaking skills.

If the size of the mount is small, then the person is inclined to be laid-back which may prove to be an obstacle in his professional life. This person will lack adequate confidence and the feeling of inferiority may easily creep in. But they are likely to have unique taste and choice. He or she will have the incessant need to be the centre of attraction. Such a person is also likely to have a hidden talent. They may indulge in a specific area of interest which may be anything like collecting antiques or food and have a passion for it. A small or flat mount of Jupiter indicates stubborn nature and a habit of flaunting what they have.

If the mount of Jupiter is inclined towards the end of the palm rather than being under the index finger the person will be insecure and self-centred, which may make him insensitive towards the feelings of others. If the mount of Jupiter is placed towards the finger of Saturn, the person will be caring and possessive. They will have a high level of intelligence with an exceptionally sharp memory.

ASTRO ADVICE

To control Jupiter, you are advised to recite the following mantra 108 times in the morning: *Aum gran grien gron sai: gurvey nameh.*

The colours yellow, off-white and orange will boost your confidence.

Pukhraj is to be worn on Thursday morning on the index finger after pran pratishtha. The weight of the stone should be according to your age and profession. It is suggested that you seek the advice of an astrologer. Wrong weight of the stone can negatively affect your career.

Donation: Donate chane ki daal on Thursday.

❖

The Mount of Saturn

The mount of Saturn is located below the longest finger of the hand which is the middle finger. This mount can influence the personality of an individual in two different ways. The person can either be overly loving and affectionate or excessively detached Similarly, the person may either have a huge social circle with an active social life or he may be a loner who dislikes socializing and prefers to be by himself.

This mount is the least noticeable mount on the hand. It is usually flat and may rarely be raised like the other mounts. If the size of this mount is overly large, then the person is likely to be self-centred. He may also be prone to depression and have a negative view towards life. Such a person does not accept defeats easily and may react rashly afterwards. He is prone to mood swings and may get angry easily due to which he may face problems in his personal relationships.

If the mount is the least prominent one, then these people are likely to be meticulous and will be very determined towards what they want to achieve. They are analytical which may help them professionally. They are extremely dutiful personally and professionally. They are likely to become ideal parents and will be extremely committed to their family life. They have a tendency to be independent from an early age and will face the hardships of life with strength and courage. They will experience success at an early age but will face a lot of struggle. They can be extremely distrustful and suspicious in their personal and professional relationships which may also make them over-possessive.

If the mount is well developed, then the person will have keen interest in law, science, history and philosophy. They can be revolutionary provided there is a reason for it. They may not always be able to express their feelings to their lovers but will show it in their actions. They prove to be loving and caring partners but may also feel insecure in relationships.

If the mount of Saturn is located towards the ring finger then the person is likely to be more expressive and sociable. They may be outgoing and will be able to communicate well with people around them. If this mount is placed towards the index finger, the person is likely to be generous, dominating and fiercely independent.

This mount reflects the general nature of a person in terms of reliability. If the mount is flat then the person will be undependable in relationships and will have a tendency to be selfish. If the mount is raised, the person will be loyal and giving in relationships.

ASTRO ADVICE

To minimize negativity, it is suggested that you recite the following mantra 108 times in the morning: *Aum aien hrin sri: shancharye nameh.*

The colours black, grey, dark brown or blue will boost your confidence.

Neelam and varieties of dark sapphire are to be worn on Thursday morning on index finger after pran pratishtha. The weight of the stone should be according to your age and profession. It is suggested that you seek the advice of an astrologer. Wrong weight of the stone can negatively affect your career.

Donation: Donate sabut dal on Saturday.

❖

The Mount of Apollo

This mount is located below the ring finger or the Apollo finger. The mount of Apollo represents the creative and artistic instinct in a person and is also known as the mount of the sun. If it is adequately raised in size, it provides a person with happiness, success and satisfaction. People who possess a well-developed mount of Apollo generally prove to be good businessmen. They are also financially blessed due to their wise and sharp character traits. Though they may be shrewd professionally, they are also fun loving.

They generally possess an eye for beauty and have a sophisticated sense of taste. Their love for beauty may sometimes prove expensive for them and they can be extravagant. They will be at their best behaviour socially and will go the extra mile to stand out in the crowd. This mount influences the person in a way that the happiness and contentment of his close ones become immensely important to him.

If the mount is higher than normal in size, the person is likely to be in search of recognition and power. They will strive to achieve name and fame. They have luxurious habits. They live for the moment, which may put them in a fix at times. They desire to possess the best of everything and work sincerely to do so but this can jeopardize their personal relationships. They have a tendency to be fake in their pursuit to be at their best behaviour at all times. They can impress a lot of people but are unlikely to touch somebody's heart easily. Because of this, they may face problems finding a partner for themselves.

If the mount is small or unnoticeable, the person will lack creativity and will be less imaginative. They will not be interested in any form of art. They also generally lack emotions and empathy, and can appear to be cold and detached at times. They dream big and plan in advance what they are going to do professionally but will not be able to implement it. They seem to be determined to do something that they want to achieve but will not be able to put in adequate effort for it. Due to this trait, they may be late starters in life with respect to their career. They will also have a practical outlook towards life.

If the mount is inclined towards the middle finger, the person will be highly imaginative and will appreciate beauty. Such a person may be a poet, an artist or a writer or just an admirer of all things creative. He may have keen interest in shaping up the immature minds of young children into something unique and creative in nature.

If this mount is inclined towards the little finger, then the person will have interest in performing arts. This person may be an actor or a director. This person is likely to be famous for his creative instincts in this area. He also has a tendency to become a social activist and have a steady career.

ASTRO ADVICE

For better results, you are advised to recite the following mantra 108 times in the morning: *Aum hran hrin hron sei: suryaye nameh.*

The colours black, grey, dark brown or blue will boost your confidence.

Ruby or amber is to be worn on Thursday morning on index finger after pran pratishtha. The weight of the stone should be according to your age and profession. It is suggested that you seek the advice of an astrologer. Wrong weight of the stone can negatively affect your career.

Donation: Donate gur (jaggery) on Thursday.

❖

The Mount of Mercury

This mount is located below the little finger and is associated with communication and intellect. This mount indicates that the character of a person is fun-loving, jolly and vivacious. This person is flexible, meticulous and intelligent. A person who possesses a full mount of mercury is likely to have a large circle of friends and an extremely active social life. He will also be expressive and will have highly-developed communication skills. Therefore, this person may be a good orator and have excellent debating skills. This person may prove extremely successful in journalism and mass media.

Such persons love to be in the company of their close ones and also possess a great sense of humour which makes them loved and admired in their social circle. People love to be in their company because of their accommodating nature. Because of their shrewdness, they prove to be successful and sharp-witted businessmen. They are also keen and dedicated workers but may have to go the extra mile to achieve their goals and realize their ambitions.

If the mount of mercury is high, the person will be exceptionally good at public speaking and communication skills. The person will have a good sense of humour but may have the tendency to be dishonest and insincere in professional and personal relationships. This type of person may prove to be an extraordinary businessman because of his cunning and shrewd ways but his deceiving nature may land him in trouble more often than not.

If the mount of mercury is small in size, the person has a tendency to be cold, unloving and uncaring in personal relationships. Such persons are impractical. They lack a sense of humour and may appear to be boring at times. They are also mostly inexpressive, leading to difficulties in their professional life as well. Success does not come easily to them no matter how hard they work. Owing to their basic nature, they are likely to have more enemies than friends who will constantly try to pull them down. Their envious counterparts may prove to be the biggest obstacles in the way of their progress.

If this mount is placed towards the ring finger then the person is likely to be merry and jovial in nature. He will also have a positive outlook towards life which will enable him to pull himself out of the trickiest situations. Therefore, he will be able to conquer all odds and obstacles that come in the way of his ambition. This trait will help him glide through the rough times. But, at the same time, the person will tend to be reckless which will work to his disadvantage.

If the mount is placed towards the end of the hand then the person will possess immense strength and courage to face the difficult times in his life. This person will be admired for his guts.

ASTRO ADVICE

For positive results, you are advised to recite the following mantra 108 times in the morning: *Aum bran brin bron se: budhaye nameh.*

The colour green will boost your confidence.

Silver and gold are to be worn on Thursday morning on index finger after pran pratishtha. It is suggested that you seek the advice of an astrologer.

Donation: Donate moongi sabut on Wednesday.

❖

Mount of Venus

This mount is formed at the base of the thumb and is encircled by the lifeline. This mount signifies love, energy and liveliness. It is associated with our ability to emotionally connect with the deeper meaning of life. It is generally regarded as the most important and vital mount of all as it influences the other mounts as well. This mount helps us know the equation of a person with his lover.

The colour of this mount also plays a significant role in informing us about the life of a person. If the colour of the mount is light pink, the person is likely to have a warm and loving nature and will have a strong sex drive. A person whose mount of Venus is pale will have a normal love and sex life with no major obstacles. A person whose mount of Venus is dark pink in colour is likely to be short-tempered and will be cold in his sex life, which may leave his partner emotionally and physically discontented. A normal-sized mount also signifies love for luxury and a lavish lifestyle.

If the mount of Venus is wide, then the person will be empathetic, broad-minded and liberal. The person will also be extremely caring and attached to his close ones and will work to maintain harmony in his relations.

If the mount of Venus is not wide or when the lifeline is closer to the thumb, then the person will be boring, calculative, selfish and inclined to have various affairs in his life.

If this mount is high, then the person will be faithful and dedicated in personal relationships. This type of person is also friendly, social and warm. The person will be highly passionate about sex and his sex life will be the dominating factor in his love life. This person will have a comfortable and lush lifestyle and will work hard to achieve it. Family life will be extremely important and a priority for this person, but he will be moody in nature which may make it difficult for people around him.

If this mount is flat, then the person will be emotionally and sexually cold. The sex drive of the person will therefore be low. This mount is considered vital as it has the strength to influence other mounts. Therefore, a flat mount can lower the positive aspects of the other mounts. The person may face an unstable love life but a stable affair can increase the size of this mount thereby lowering the negativity related to the flat mount.

ASTRO ADVICE

In order to improve your love life you are advised to recite the following mantra 108 times in the morning: *Aum hran hrin hron sei: shukraye nameh.*

The colours blue and royal blue will boost your confidence.

Diamond or Sapphire is to be worn on Thursday morning on index finger after pran pratishtha. The weight of the stone should be according to your age and profession. It is suggested you seek the advice of an astrologer. Wrong weight of the stone can negatively affect your life.

Donation: Donate milk on Monday.

❖

Mount of Mars

There are two mounts of Mars; one is the upper mars and the other is lower Mars. The lower Mars is located between the mount of Jupiter and the mount of Venus or between the index finger and the thumb. The upper Mars is located opposite the thumb, between the head and the heart line.

Both the mounts have unique characteristics. The lower Mars signifies physical strength and stamina in a person. It reveals the level of assertiveness in a person. On the other hand, the upper Mars indicates the inner strength and willpower in a person. Both these are similar in some aspects and totally opposite to each other in certain others.

Lower Mount of Mars

This is the small amount of skin which gathers together when the thumb makes a movement. It represents the amount of power a person possesses to face an adverse situation. It combines mental strength with physical strength. A person whose mount is normal-sized will be courageous enough to face tricky situations and stand up for himself.

If this mount is small in size, it signifies that the person will lack the strength to deal with tough situations. He will be dependent or cowardly in nature.

If this mount is large, then the person will be fearless to the extent of being fierce. The person will be cold in nature and will be indifferent towards the feelings of others. He will have the tendency to be short-tempered and moody which makes it extremely difficult to deal with him.

Upper Mount of Mars

The role of this mount is considered to be passive. The heart line usually starts where this mount ends opposite the thumb. This mount provides a person with energy, power, perseverance and strength of mind. A person with upper mount of Mars that is normal in size will be mentally balanced and will not be aroused easily at an aggravation. He will have the ability to think before he acts. He is very tactful in personal and professional relationships.

If this mount is small in size then the person will be inexpressive and unpredictable. He can either be extremely calm or short-tempered. He does not take criticism sportingly and may become defensive when criticized.

If this mount is big, the person will have the tendency to be very determined, to the extent of being obsessive. They are cold and dominating. They are likely to be harsh.

ASTRO ADVICE

To boost your level of endurance you are advised to recite the following mantra 108 times in the morning: *Aum hran hrin hron sai angaarkaye nameh.*

The colours red, orange and white will boost your confidence.

Coral (moonga) is to be worn on Thursday morning on index finger after pran pratishtha. The weight of the stone should be according to your age and profession. It is suggested you seek the advice of an astrologer. Wrong weight of the stone can negatively affect your career and your life.

Donation: Donate wheat on Thursday.

❖

Mount of Luna

The mount of Luna is that part of the hand which is located opposite the thumb, starting from the wrist towards the little finger. This mount relates to the softer side of a person's character. It reflects the emotional instinct of a person. It also provides insight into the creative side of an individual.

It helps us to know the romantic side of a person. If this mount is the most prominent mount, the person is likely to be a good planner but will lack the initiative to put his plan into action. Such a person will have a very casual view towards life and be fake; he or she will be polite and well-mannered outwardly but lack feeling within.

If this mount is high, the person is likely to be a day-dreamer and therefore inclined to take wrong decisions in life. Such a person will be childish and immature. He will have a love for travelling and is likely to choose a profession that involves travelling. He is also prone to anxiety and may be full of energy. He lacks a realistic attitude and will mostly aim for goals that are impossible to achieve and will end up spending endless energy and time on it.

If this mount is small, the person lacks emotion and is likely to be indifferent towards the feelings of others. Such a person may not be faithful and trustworthy and is, therefore, likely to have more foes than friends. This person will have an eye for detail, with a tendency to be finicky about minute things which may be annoying for the people around him. He may prove to be a good worker in his profession.

The travel lines are also present in the mount of Moon but the size of the mount plays a vital role in determining the outcome of these lines. If the size of the mount is large, the person will be restless and inclined to travel very often. Such a person would love to visit new places and learn about various cultures. If the size of the mount is small and there is the presence of travel lines, the person will be inclined to travelling comfortably, but will be fond of it nevertheless.

ASTRO ADVICE

To improve your communication skills you are adivised to recite the following mantra 108 times in the morning: *Aum shran shrin shron se: chandraye nameh.*

The colours white, light yellow and sea colour will boost your confidence.

Pearl or cat's eye is to be worn on Thursday morning on index finger after pran pratishtha. The weight of the stone should be according to your age and profession. It is suggested you seek the advice of an astrologer. Wrong weight of the stone can negatively affect your career and your life.

Donation: Donate rice on Monday.

Mount of Neptune

This mount is not very common. It is located at the base of the hand, just above the wrist. It is situated between the mount of Venus and the mount of Luna.

A fully developed mount of Neptune makes a person a good orator with extraordinary communication skills. It makes a person spontaneous. It is mostly found in the hands of politicians, leaders, actors and performers.

If this mount is of the same size as the mounts of Luna and Venus, the person will be ambitious in nature and is most likely to be successful professionally. Such a person will also be a sociable in nature.

ASTRO ADVICE

For a positive effect you are advised to recite the following mantra for 108 times in the morning: *Aum shran shrin shron se: chandraye nameh.*

The colours white, light yellow and sea colour will boost your confidence.

Pearl or cat's eye is to be worn on Thursday morning on index finger after pran pratishtha. The weight of the stone should be according to your age and profession. It is suggested you seek the advice of an astrologer. Wrong weight of the stone can negatively affect your career and your life.

Donation: Donate rice on Monday.

8

Major Lines

INTRODUCTION

The lines on a hand are the most prominent and vital part of palmistry. They are the foremost thing people relate to in palmistry. These lines are like an index to the story of the life of a person. They disclose all the facts about all the spheres of a person's life which relate to his past, present or future. These lines change from time to time, therefore, the outcome is never static but can change according to a person's virtues and vices.

There are mainly four major lines on the hand; the heart, head, life and destiny line. The shape of the hand, the fingers and the nails collectively play an important role in determining a person's past, present and future. Each line reveals something different about his/her life.

The heart line helps us know about an individual's personal life and his love life.

The lifeline helps us to know about a person's health, physical fitness and stamina. Unlike what is generally believed, the lifeline not only determines how long a person will live, but also relates to the physical strength of a person.

The head line tells us about the thought process of a person. It helps us to know the mentality of a person which is extremely vital in knowing about his/her character.

The destiny line helps us to know the direction of a person's life. It guides us towards the objective of a person's life. It reveals the main reason that instills a driving spirit in a person.

All these lines together constitute the vital aspects of a person's life. Ideally, all these lines should be clear, indicating a hassle-free life. The lines should also be prominent, and the deeper they are marked, the stronger will their significance be in our lives. Weak lines indicate lesser significance and influence in our lives. At times even the lighter markings, which are not clearly visible, can make a difference. At the same time, if a person has very few lines on his hand, it does not necessarily mean that the person will have an exceptionally good life. Such a person may also lead a very simple and ordinary life.

One hand is the hand of potential and the other is the active hand. The hand of potential signifies our past and the active hand signifies our present and future. If the hand of potential depicts an unclear and uneven lifeline and the active hand shows a more prominent lifeline, it denotes that the person has conquered the problems in his life. In some cases, the hand of potential is clearer than the active hand; then the active hand will indicate the reason for interruption that caused changes in the person's life after a good beginning.

THE LIFELINE

The lifeline is considered to be the most significant line on the hand. It is the only line related to almost all the vital aspects of life. Every line on the hand, other than the lifeline, is related to the information that this line provides. It is like an index of the life of an individual.

It is generally believed that the lifeline foretells the span of our existence. It is only a myth that a short lifeline necessarily means a short life and a long one denotes a long life. This line is the most misunderstood line of all.

This line is located between the thumb and the index finger or the Jupiter finger. It starts almost half-way between the two, forms a semi circle and encircles the thumb and finishes almost where the wrist starts or a little before in certain cases. If the semicircle is large in size, then it signifies that the person will have immense enthusiasm and strength. Such a person will be daring, fun-loving and courageous. If it is small, the person will lack direction in life and will have a low level of energy. This line encircles the mount of Venus which rests at the base of the thumb.

The lifeline indicates power, strength and vitality in a person. If the line is strong as well as long, it indicates that the person will have immense energy, zest and stamina. It also relates to the level of passion in a person and therefore the level of satisfaction and happiness in a person's life. Each lifeline will be different from the other, no matter how similar they seem at first. There are bound to be differences but the basic arrangement of the line will be the same. An interruption in this line does not necessarily mean something negative. It may indicate a change in the direction of life in terms of profession or relationships.

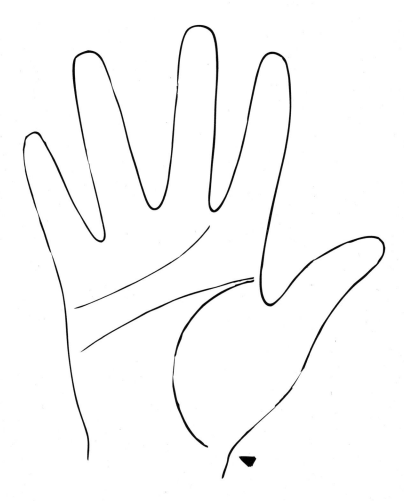

The Lifeline

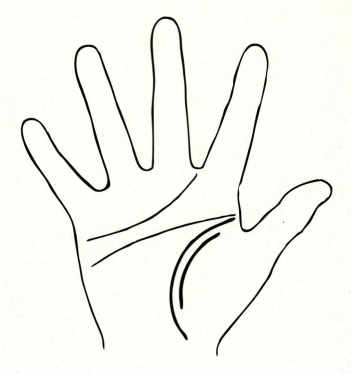

Sister Line (Also known as the Line of Mars)

A line may or may not be uniform throughout. It may start very clearly, become lighter towards the middle and end on a clearer note. In such cases, it means that the person had a loss of sense of direction somewhere in between, where his level of enthusiasm was lower compared to the rest of his life. As I mentioned earlier, a person's lifeline should ideally be neat without any minor lines and markings, as well as deep. Such a line means you will have an enthusiastic approach towards life and it indicates physical well-being of the person.

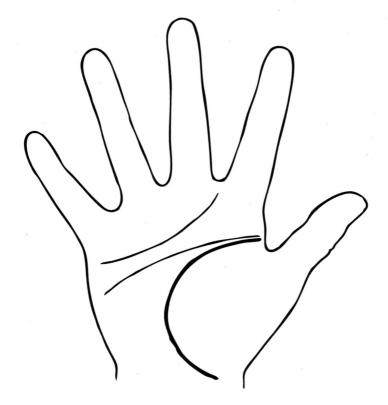

Lifeline Coming well across the Palm Energy

If there is a gap in the lifeline, it suggests that the person had a change of interest or his life's perspective took a drastic turn which may have been due to ill health or change of relationships. These gaps tend to form a small extra line which fills the gap called a 'sister line'.

The sister line forms in the semicircle on the hand. This line runs alongside the lifeline and is shorter than the lifeline. This line mitigates the negative effects of the gap in the lifeline. The more prominent part of the sister line implies that during that period, the problems occurring due to the gap were balanced by the sister line and vice versa. Therefore, the presence of this line is always positive.

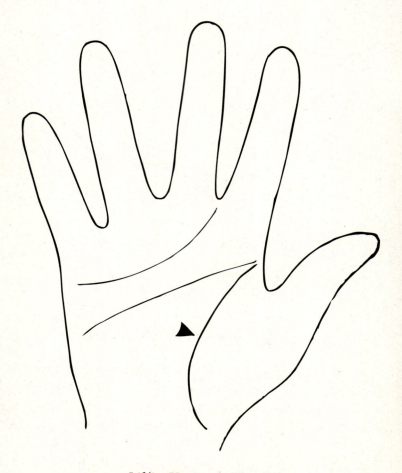

Lifeline Hugging the Thumb

SEGMENTS OF THE LIFELINE

The First Quarter

The lifeline begins between the thumb and the index finger. An irregular beginning of this line implies that the person had a below-average beginning in his life. It implies ill health during childhood or unhappiness during adolescent years. If the line begins from a curve in the beginning and there are gaps in the initial part of the line, it means that the person had an unconventional birth. The first quarter of the lifeline, which tells us about the first quarter of our life, is mainly about the parent-child relationship.

The Second Quarter

This quarter foretells about the life from twenty-five to fifty years. If the arc of this part of life is well formed, sans any gaps and irregularities, it indicates a level-headed approach towards life. It denotes that the person has the sense to weigh the pros and cons of each situation before taking any step forward. He moves in life with a firm objective and has a definite sense of direction. If there are small lines attached to the lifeline in this segment, it means that an extra effort was made during that period to accomplish goals and objectives. If the line is close to the thumb, it signifies a stable and ordinary life. This denotes a steady, average, and to some extent, a dull life. If the lifeline passes midway through the palm it means that the person will have an interesting and extraordinary life. He will have an urge for independence and enthusiasm to try new things in life. He will strongly oppose a static and monotonous way of life and will constantly strive for change.

The Last Quarter

If the line ends prominently and is long, it signifies that the person will have sound health during the last quarter of his life. Such a person is likely to be active and involved in social work during his old age. He will take interest in leisurely activities and will be lively even at that stage in life. Various lines on and around the lifeline imply that there has been deterioration in the physical and mental state of the person over the years.

If a person has a lifeline that touches the wrist and is clear towards the end, it means that the person loves to travel even if it is to nearby places.

MARKINGS ON THE LIFELINE

Squares

The effect of a square on the lifeline depends on where it is located. Its effect may not necessarily be positive or negative. For instance, if a square covers a gap, then it means that the square minimizes the negative effect caused by that gap. A gap usually means loss of direction, disturbance in career or ill health. When a square covers such a gap, it implies that such difficulty in life stands evaded, or its outcome minimized. It instils courage and strength to deal with the problem.

If there is a square over a part of the lifeline that does not have any gap, it indicates unhappiness. It means that during this period the person had restrictions and did not have the freedom to fulfil his desires. It could mean the restrictions were either imposed or the person lacked the resources to fulfil them. It may mean the person has been or will be imprisoned during that phase but it may also mean he had no power or authority to exercise his will.

A square may appear and disappear with time as lines and markings keep changing according to the deeds of a person. It is eventually the person himself who controls his destiny and not vice versa.

Worry Lines

These lines start from the base of the thumb and advance towards the lifeline, sometimes even cross them. A person who has numerous worry lines will be pessimistic and overly anxious. Having many worry lines may not necessarily mean that the person will have problematic life as the worry may also be a trait of the person.

If the worry lines cross the lifeline it may negatively influence a person's physical state. Therefore, I believe having a positive state of mind and diverting the mind towards peaceful activities like social work, religious affairs and yoga can bring down the anxiety level of a person. This can lower the effect of worry lines.

ASTRO ADVICE

For longevity, remedies of Jupiter and Saturn should be taken. You are advised to recite the following mantra 108 times in the morning: *Aum gran grien gron sai: gurvey nameh.*

The colour white, light yellow and black will boost your confidence.

Pukhraj and Neelam are to be worn on Thursday morning on index finger after pran pratishtha. The weight of the stone should be according to your age and profession. It is suggested you seek the advice of an astrologer. Wrong weight of the stone can negatively affect your career and your life.

Donation: Donate maa sabut and chane ki daal on Saturday.

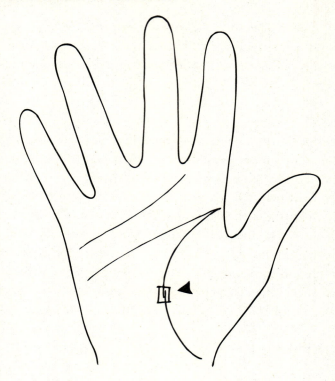

Protective Square on the Lifeline

HEAD LINE

After observing the lifeline, let us study the head line. It indicates a person's intellectual level and the way a person executes his intellect. It starts between the thumb and the first finger. It tells us about the mental ability of a person. It also tells us about the career path and how a person deals with various circumstances in his life. If a person possesses a good lifeline but at the same time a weak head line, it means that the person will have many good opportunities in life but will not be able to make full use of them.

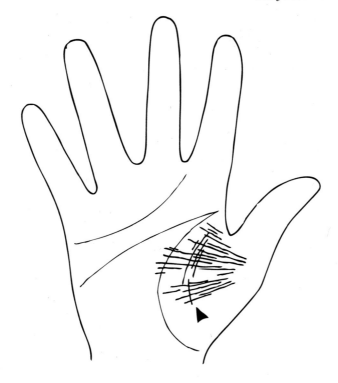

Worry Lines

As is the case with the lifeline, a person's head line should ideally be clear, well marked and free of any breaks or gaps. If there is any break in the head line, it means that a person is not fully utilizing his intelligence. A clear head line indicates that the person has adequate self-belief and intellect to put his thoughts into action and has self-control. It is rare to come across a perfect head line. Such a person will be career-oriented, successful and have a sense of direction in life. This type of person will possess an immensely business-oriented mind with a strong intuitive quality in matters of profession. The length of the head line does not make much of

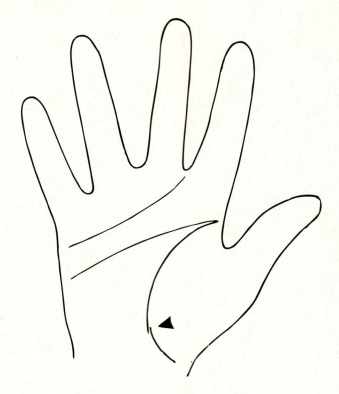

Break in Lifeline

a difference, as a long or short head line does not necessarily mean anything positive or negative.

At times when a head line is weak, a strong mercury line affects it in a positive way and minimizes the negative effect. Similarly, if the top end of the thumb is straight, then it denotes confidence and a sense of security which prove useful to the person professionally.

A flat head line means that the person is humble by nature, has tremendous level of concentration, but lacks creativity. A person

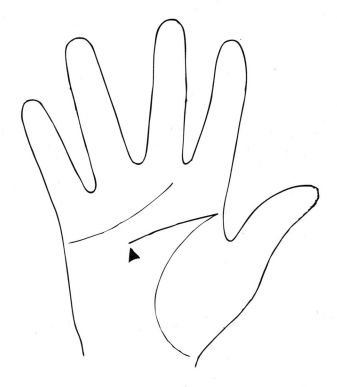

Head Line

whose head line is curved towards the base of the hand is likely to be more creative and shrewd. This type of person may be an actor, an artist, a writer or a poet. At the same time, it is absolutely necessary that the person channels his creative instinct in the right direction.

Many a times, the head line ends in fork-like lines. These lines suggest a good balance between reasoning and intuition as long as they are free from any marks. This channels his creativity in the right direction with logic. A clear and strong line means that the person's reasoning power is good and he is able to tackle adverse circumstances by making the most of his intelligence.

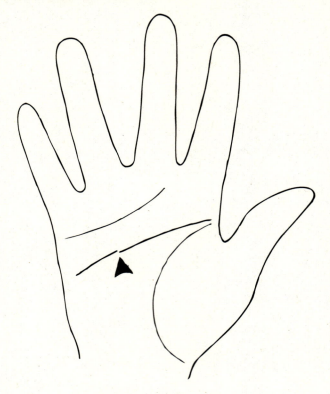

Break in the Head Line

If the head line in a person's hand is more prominent, the person will have a scholarly and studious bent of mind. A faint line does not necessarily mean that the person lacks intelligence; it signifies that the person may have an artistic bent of mind. This does not mean that person will be an under-achiever; just that the person lacks the ability to reap fruitful results of his efforts. Such a person is more likely to have problems related to blood pressure and hypertension.

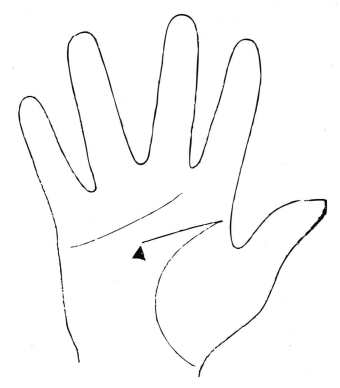

Short Head Line

If the head line is bent in the end such a person will be worldly in nature and may have luxurious habits. This type of person will be goal-oriented and will make an extra effort to fulfil his desires.

If the end of the head line splits into two, it implies that the person will have strong emotions and will have the tendency to fall in love very easily.

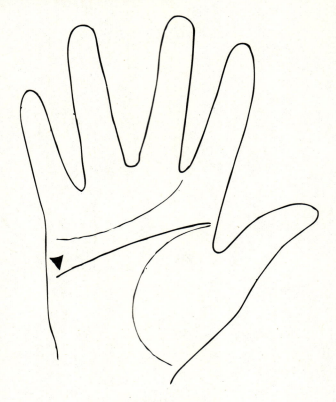

Very Long Head Line

If the head line does not touch the lifeline, a person is likely to be fun-loving, self-reliant and confident. He will live this life on the spur of the moment and follow his heart more than logic. The bigger the gap, the more outgoing and spontaneous the person will be. If the head line touches the lifeline the person will be alert and analytical in his approach. This type of person will essentially weigh the pros and cons of each situation before actually taking a decision. He has an eye for detail and is extremely cautious.

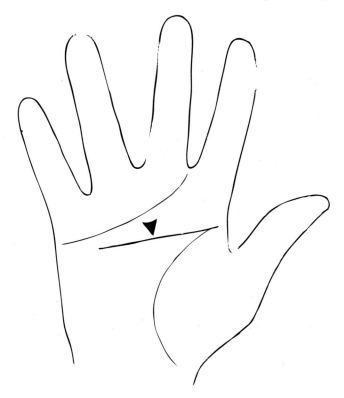

Practical Head Line

SEGMENTS OF THE HEAD LINE

First Quarter

If the head line is more prominent at the starting, then the person is likely to make better use of his reasoning skills in the later stage of his life. If a person has a long head line, it implies that the person will have a variety of interests and hobbies. A person

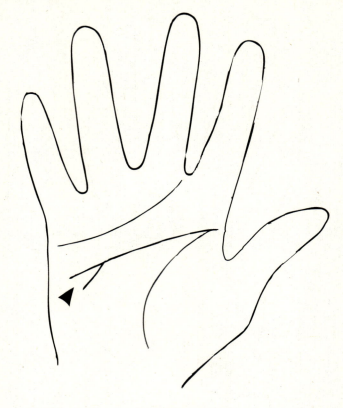

Writer's Fork

with a prominent head line at the start is likely to have a long head line. Such people have the ability to utilize each opportunity to the fullest. Therefore, they are likely to be extremely successful in their career.

They have instinctive qualities and will work timelessly towards their career and will not be disheartened easily by setbacks. Since they are backed by positivism and intelligence, nothing can stop them from what they intend to achieve. They also keep themselves occupied in their varied interests.

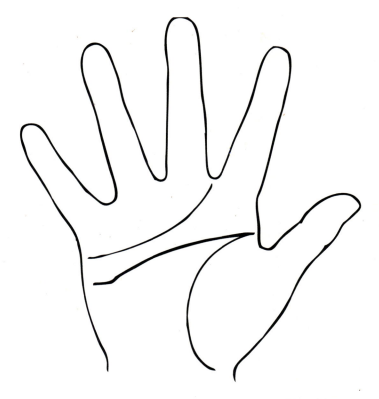

Head Line with Distinct Bend at the End (Material Needs)

Second Quarter

If the head line starts prominently and gradually becomes fainter towards the middle, it means that the person has not made optimum use of his abilities and opportunities that came his way. This could also mean that unfavourable circumstances have played spoilsport in the person's life which prove to be an obstacle in his career. Ideally, the middle part of the head line should be free of any gaps, breaks or marks. Absence of these indicates that the person has a

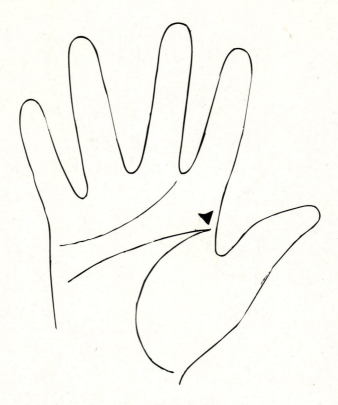

Head Line Joined to Lifeline

very smooth adult life sans any problems. This generally has the possibility of hampering a person's self-confidence.

Third Quarter

A sloping head line towards the end indicates creative instinct and an innovative bent of mind. An overly sloping line signifies that the person has an inclination towards being overly imaginative to the extent of being unreal. If there is a gap in the last quarter, it

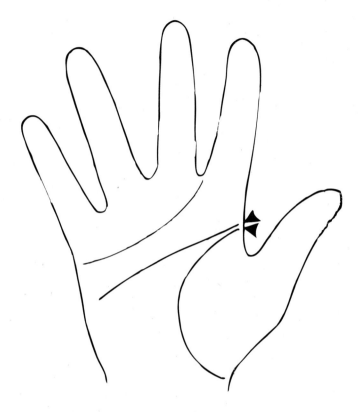

Head Line Starting Independently from the Lifeline

means that the person's reasoning power and intelligence have been affected. A weak head line in the end signifies negative effect of age on the memory and intellect of person. Similarly, a stronger head line towards the end signifies that the person's level of intelligence has not been affected by age.

ASTRO ADVICE

For optimum use of one's capabilities, remedies of Mercury should be taken. You are advised to recite the following mantra 108 times in the morning: *Aum bran brin bron se: budhaye nameh.*

The colour green will be beneficial for you.

Panna is to be worn on Wednesday morning on the little finger after pran pratishtha. The weight of the stone should be according to your age and profession. It is suggested you seek the advice of an astrologer. Wrong weight of the stone can negatively affect your career and your life.

Donation: Donate moong sabut on Wednesday.

HEART LINE

The heart line is also known as the line of imagination and it relates to the emotional state of a person. It conveys how emotionally expressive a person is. Therefore, it also tells us about a person's love life and the level of warmth in the emotions. Each person's view and capacity to love is different from the other and this line helps us to know about a person's point of view towards love and personal relationships.

This line starts beneath the little finger and goes up to the second or the third finger. It is usually classified into two types. The first type of heart line is known as the physical heart line; this line is a curve. It ends around the first and the second finger. Such people are comparatively more expressive. They have the ability to be emotionally warm and have no qualms about showing the way they feel. Hence, they have a good social circle with many people close to their heart. Personal relationships are of extreme importance to them. They will also be caring and concerned about the people around them.

The second type of heart line is known as the mental heart line and this line is flat. Such people are not very expressive. Though they are not always emotionally cold, they have a tendency to keep their feelings to themselves. This trait makes it extremely difficult for people around them to judge what they feel. Therefore, one has to be extra careful about what is said to them because if they feel hurt or offended, they will not show it. They will also be vulnerable and need constant reassurances. They may appear to be self-centred in personal relationships.

This line is most prone to change since the emotional state of a person keeps varying. Therefore, this line and the markings on it tell us a lot about the state of personal relationships in a person's life. It is favourable for one person in a relationship to have these markings, else both will be prone to friction. But even then they can have a good bonding if they learn to overcome each other's traits and value togetherness.

The heart line also conveys the state of a person's health and helps us to know about the disturbances, if any, in the health of a person. If there is any possibility of a heart problem or any other disease, it can be seen in the markings on the heart line. Even depression caused due to emotional setbacks can be observed on this line. They can be seen in the form of various small lines emerging out of the heart line.

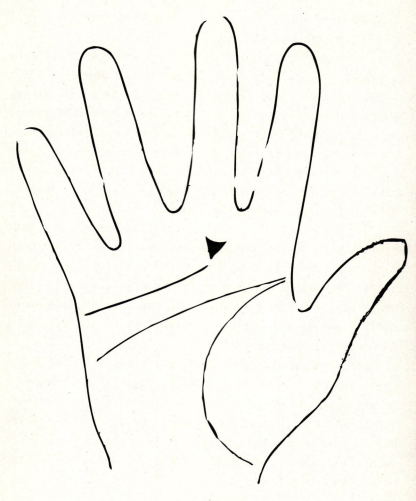

Mental Heart Line

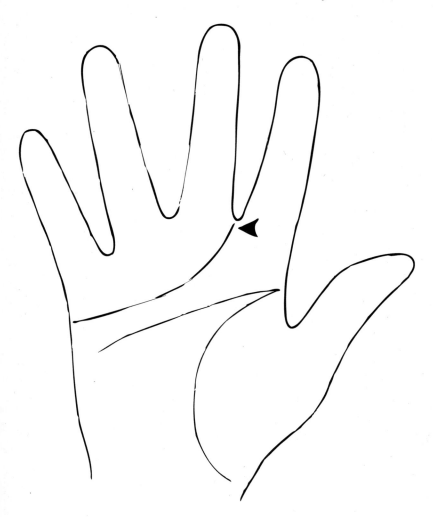

Physical Heart Line

Another vital thing to keep in mind while studying the heart line is how it ends. When the heart line ends below the first finger or the index finger, a person is likely to be sensitive and easily hurt. They are mostly very organised and likely to follow clichés. They expect their partners to reciprocate in the same way; they get disheartened easily.

If the heart line ends below the second finger then the person is likely to be dissatisfied in relationships. But this may not be the case always; the markings on the heart line can bring warmth in the person. This person has the tendency to be demanding in relationships and be self-centred.

If the heart line ends between the first and the second finger, which is very common, this person will be a blend of the above traits. He will be loving but at the same time concerned and expect love from his loved ones. He will be giving in personal relationships and at the same time want his own desires to be fulfilled as well. Such people have a practical approach towards life but at the same time have an element of emotion in them.

If the heart line ends in a fork shape, it signifies that such people have traits of both types of heart lines. This blend of traits can be positive or negative depending on the traits that they acquire from both the cases. Such people can be extremely tough and this may make it difficult for others to deal with them.

SEGMENTS OF THE HEART LINE

First Quarter

Ideally, the initial part of the heart line should be free of any gaps, moles or markings. A clear and smooth line in the beginning implies that the person has had an emotionally contented and happy childhood. But, if the heart line has any such breaks or markings, it means that the person was emotionally disturbed during his childhood.

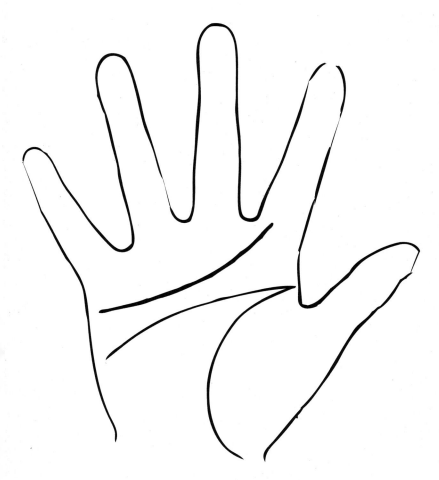

Heart Line Ending below First Finger

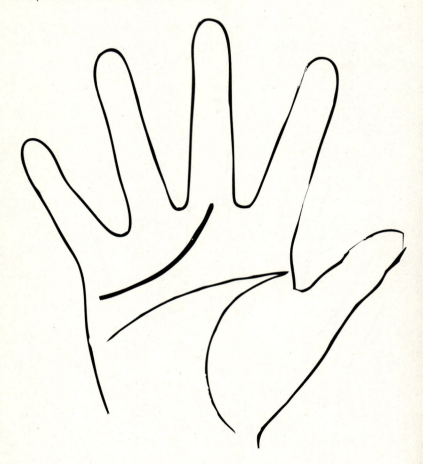

Heart Line Ending below Second Finger

If the heart line, lifeline and head line are all joined together at the start, the person will be successful in all aspects of his life. Such a person will have firm determination and tend to achieve his goals. High placement of heart line signifies that the person has a strong intuitive power. This type of person will also have a blissful life.

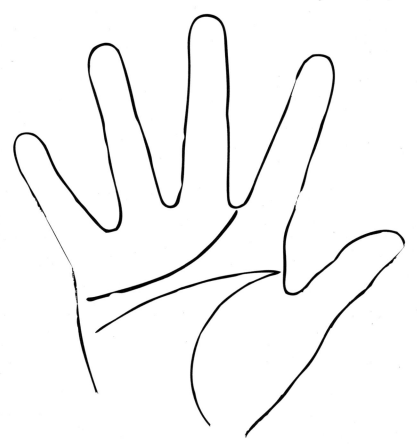

Heart Line Ending between First and Second Fingers

Second Quarter

This is the most active and vital section of the heart line since it denotes the young age where emotions play a dominant role in life. If there is a gap in this period it implies that the person will be emotionally stressed or disturbed. It can also mean that the person's health will suffer in this period.

If the line is more prominent during this period, it means that the person's emotions are extremely active and that he enjoys a good love life during this period. Similarly, a faint heart line during this period means that the person is on quest for love but is not successful.

Third Quarter

If there is a fork-like ending of the heart line where it splits into three sections, it means that the person will be able to manage his emotions in a very balanced and stable way. This means that the emotional state of the person during the last stage of his life is indeed positive.

A low-lying heart line means that the person will be extremely possessive of his close ones, especially his lover. This possessive attitude could also take the form of envy or suspicion and create a rift in the relationship. Such persons enjoy luxury and will make every effort to have a comfortable and lavish lifestyle.

ASTRO ADVICE

For optimum use of one's capabilities, remedies of Mercury should be taken. You are advised to recite the following mantra 108 times in the morning: *Aum bran brin bron se: budhaye nameh.*

The colour green will be beneficial for you.

Neelam or Pukhraj is to be worn on Thursday morning on the index finger after pran pratishtha. The weight of the stone should be according to your age and profession. It is suggested you seek the advice of an astrologer. Wrong weight of the stone can negatively affect your career and your life.

Donation: Donate moongi sabut and chane ki daal on Wednesday.

The Fate Line

This line is also known as the line of Saturn and not everyone possesses this line. The word 'fate' refers to the happenings in the entire lifetime. This line is situated in the middle of the palm starting near the wrist and ending towards the fingers. The fate line starts near the head or lifeline and at times even touches them. The position of the other lines does not vary as much as the position of the fate line.

A strong destiny line indicates that there are more chances of the person having greater accomplishments in life. This line helps us to know to what extent a person's career aspirations are achieved. This line has a major positive effect on the career of a person. The formation of this also depends on our childhood and our state of mind during these early years. At times, the fate line begins near the head line; it means the person did not have a sense of direction professionally and only at the stage where the fate line began, he realised the direction of his career.

Sometimes the destiny line is virtually non-existent until the twenties or even thirties. A weak fate line in between implies that the career path that the person has chosen is not what he intended to do. It means that the person's current profession is something he chose due to family pressure or circumstances. A person may be well established in his current career but a weak fate line indicates the above circumstances.

A clear and smooth fate line means that the person will never be out of job and have a smooth career sans any obstacles. Such a person is also inclined to devote several years of service in one job.

If such a line exists on the palm of a woman who is a housewife, it means she will enjoy a blissful marriage and a comfortable life at home and feel content in her life.

If the line is not clear or uneven, it means that the person is not satisfied with his career. Similarly, if a woman who is a housewife has a broken fate line, it implies she is not satisfied in the conventional role. She has the urge to do something more in her life.

Breaks in one part of the line and a smooth formation in the other denotes that at the stage where the smooth fate line began the person realized his goal in life. If initially the line is uneven and later smooth, it means that the person had no sense of direction in the initial part of his life. If the fate line is smooth in the beginning and then tends to become uneven, it means that the person had ambition in the initial stage of his life but with the passing of years, he has had a loss of direction.

This line indicates that the person has a set goal in his life that he wants to achieve. It indicates a driving spirit in a person regarding his career. This instils determination in a person to attain his goal. Such people have a clear fate line that is free of any marks or breaks. The existence of fate line signifies that the person will have the inclination to take the right decisions regarding his career.

But, if this line is the most prominent line on the palm it means that the person has a tendency to overwork and hardly has any time left for family or friends. This could leave him feeling empty at times.

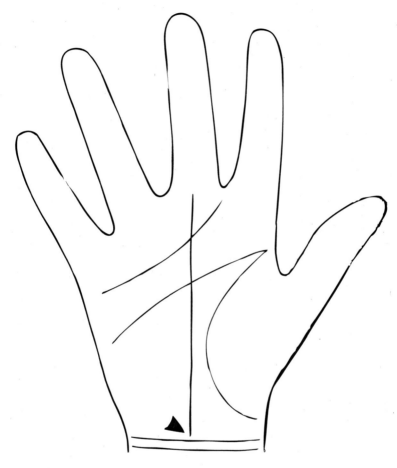

Destiny Line

A weak fate line implies instability or dissatisfaction in the career path. It also means that the profession that the person has currently chosen is not what that person intended to do.

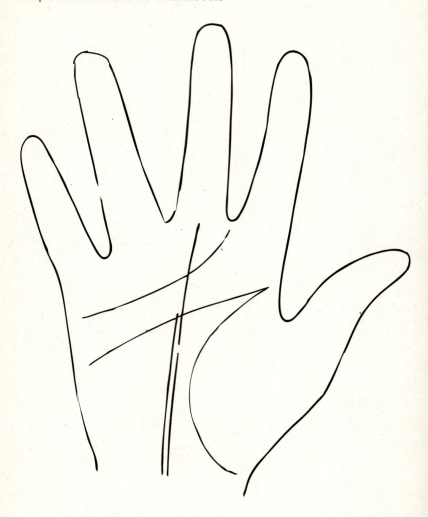

Break in Destiny Line

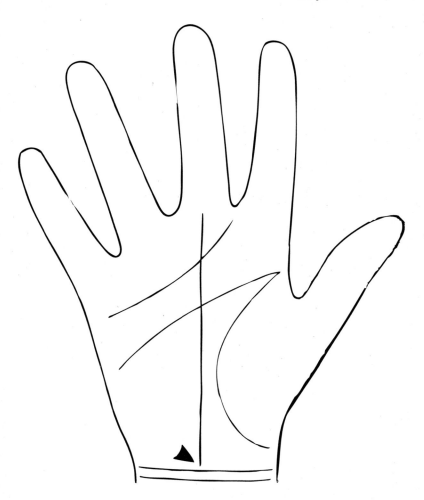

Destiny Line Starting Early in Life

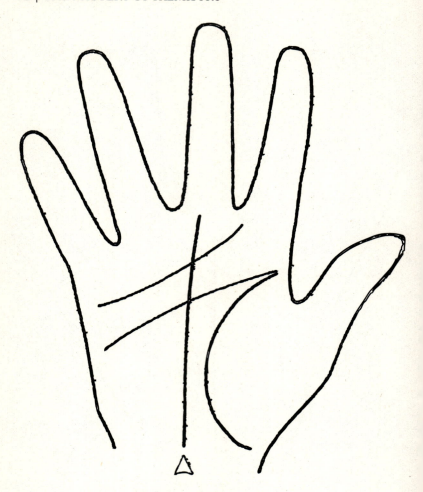

Independent Start to Destiny Line

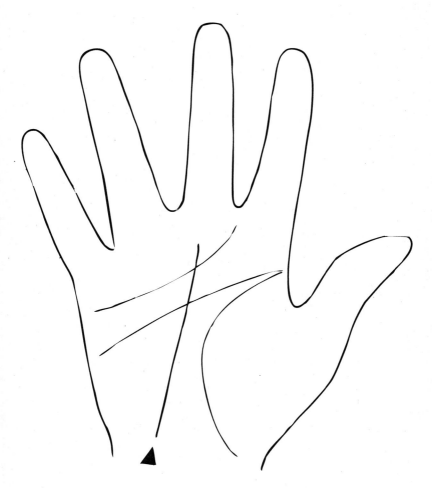

Destiny Line Starting well across the Palm

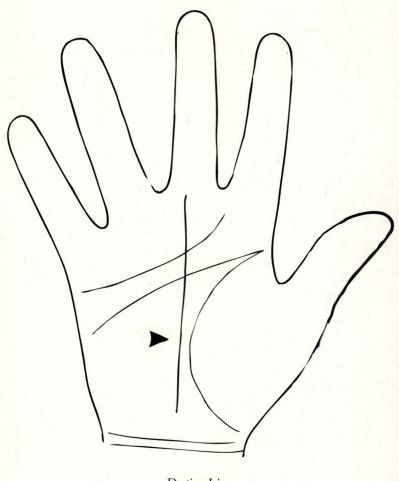

Destiny Line

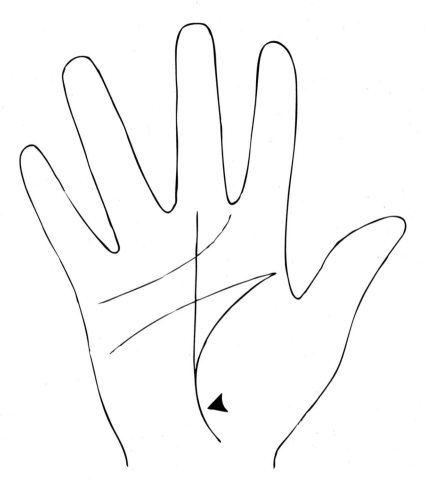

Destiny Line Attached to Lifeline

SEGMENTS OF THE FATE LINE

First Segment

The first section of the fate line tells us about those years when the person tries to decide the direction of his life. If this part of the fate line is smooth sans any breaks, it signifies that the person has had a good education. Though it does not indicate about the personal life of that individual, a good educational background signifies a positive role of the family in the person's life.

Gaps or breaks in the initial stage of the fate line indicate that the person was unsure about the career he wanted to pursue and recurrent changes in the direction he is to follow. It means that the person had various career options in mind and his choices kept fluctuating. An even fate line in the beginning tells us that the person had a firm idea of what he wanted to become in his life since childhood. But, gradually, if a person's fate line forms into a smooth line after various gaps then it means that the person finally decided which direction he wanted to pursue in his life. The point from where this smooth line starts determines at what stage the person realized his goal in life.

Second Segment

This is the most vital section in a person's fate line since it is here the formation of a person's career actually takes shape. This is the stage where a person builds his career and the efforts are rewarded. Out of all the segments, it is most important for this section to be smooth as the success and failure of a person's career is mainly determined by this period in a person's life. At times, there is a break in the fate line which indicates a change of direction or career in life. When the gap in the break is large, it indicates that there was a break in the career of the person which could be because he left the job, was dismissed or a disappointment in life made him drift from his goals and ambitions.

Third Segment

Usually, in the third and last segment of the fate line, it tends to fade and become less prominent. Similarly, if the fate line is short in length or we can say if the last stage of the person's fate line is missing, it means that the person has taken an early retirement. The fate line is rarely prominent in this stage. In such a case, it means that the person has chosen a new career option in his retirement age which provides him success and contentment.

If there are several breaks in the fate line at this stage, it indicates disharmony in the life of the person. If there are several minor lines attached to this line during this stage, it signifies that the person has taken up various activities to keep himself busy and utilize time.

ASTRO ADVICE

For fulfillment of goals and desires, remedies of Mercury should be taken. You are advised to recite the following mantra 108 times in the morning: *Aum aien hrin sri: shancharye nameh.*

The colours black, grey, dark brown or blue will be beneficial for you.

Neelam or varieties of dark saphhire should be worn on Thursday morning on index finger after pran pratishtha. The weight of the stone should be in accordance with your age and profession. It is suggested you seek the advice of an astrologer. Wrong weight of the stone can negatively affect your career and your life.

Donation: Donate maa sabut on Saturday.

THE APOLLO LINE

The Apollo line, also known as the Line of the Sun, can be termed as the second fate line. This line greatly influences the fate line. In case a person has a weak fate line and a strong line of sun sans any markings or breaks, then the Line of the Sun minimizes the negative effects of a weak fate line. Ideally, it should be long, clear and free of any marks. This line, if perfect in its formation, has a positive effect on every other line on the palm.

It starts from the direction of the wrist and advances towards the third or the ring finger. This line when perfect in shape indicates a comfortable and fortunate life. It enhances the chances of success and achievement of aspirations. Mostly, it is not very prominent in nature and is essentially the line of contentment. A strong fate line signifies success in career and accomplishment of goals but it does not necessarily mean that the person is happy; whereas the presence of the Line of the Sun necessarily means that the person is happy with his life and satisfied with his level of achievement.

This line does not essentially indicate achievements and professional success. It may also mean that the person has acquired a comfortable living by birth or by inheritance. People who have unique tastes and talent like a person who is an actor, an artist or a musician, usually have this line. They are also seen in those people who establish their career based on an unusual choice or direction. They are creative and bold and stand up for what they believe in.

If this line is short, it indicates that the person will not be able to achieve much in life even though he may possess the capacity. This line should be long, clear and free of gaps to be considered fortunate. It is not only considered auspicious financially but also bestows a blissful life without any major setbacks and problems.

This line may be perceived auspicious only in terms of money, but it is not necessary for the person to be rich. It may mean an ordinary life in which all the needs and comforts of the person are taken care of. In such a case, the person is not dissatisfied with life and is pleased with the way he is leading his life. Therefore, this line has got to do more with inner happiness and material achievements.

In case this line is very faint, it means that the person makes optimum efforts in life but the appreciation of his efforts is absent. Such a person lives his life without getting noticed much and without being valued for his work.

Length of the Apollo Line

A long and well-established Apollo line with less or no breaks in between signifies that the person has been focused towards his goal in life since the very start. It means furthermore that with advancing of years, the person has made enough efforts to achieve what he intended to. A long or full fate line indicates that the person has lived a successful and content professional life.

A short Apollo line means that the person was carrying out his career objectives successfully, but along the way the person's career came to a halt due to a personal or professional setback. In such cases, a person only advances further in his career after he has been motivated by inner or outer forces to move on in life. A short fate line is also present in cases where a person has over-achieved in his career, and has enough resources to spend the rest of his life without making any more efforts. This is a case where the person retires earlier than expected.

STARTING POSITION OF THE APOLLO LINE

Starting From Lifeline

If a person's Apollo line is close to his lifeline, it indicates that this type of person loves being in the company of his close ones and does not prefer being alone. Therefore, such persons are inclined to work and perform better in groups. Such people are overly protective and possessive about their loved ones. They are likely to have been influenced in a positive way while growing up due to family bonding and warmth in relationships. Such people will always prioritize near ones over everything else in life.

Starting From the Centre of the Palm

When a person's Apollo line starts from the base of the palm and crosses the centre of the palm, such a person will be fiercely independent. This could be because of his circumstances during childhood. A person may have studied in a boarding school or may have become an orphan at an early age. They will not be intimidated by others and will have the courage to stand up for themselves and for what they want in life.

ASTRO ADVICE

For optimum use of one's capabilities, suggestive remedies of Sun should be taken. You are advised to recite the following mantra 108 times in the morning: *Aum hran hrin hron sei: suryaye nameh.*

The colours red, orange and white will be beneficial for you.

Ruby or amber is to be worn on Thursday morning on the index finger after pran pratishtha. The weight of the stone should be according to your age and profession. It is suggested you seek the advice of an astrologer. Wrong weight of the stone can have adverse effects on your career life.

Donation: Donate jaggery on Sunday.

9

Minor Lines

Minor lines are those which are not very prominent but are significant and therefore, their meaning and the purpose of their existence should be known.

Many of these lines are only stress lines and therefore not all of them are significant. Ideally, a person should have lesser number of lines on his palm, but certain minor lines are auspicious and have a positive influence on our lives.

THE INTUITION LINE

This line is a semicircle which begins from the Lunar mount, crosses the middle of the palm, and extends up to the mount of Mercury. This line instils the power of intuition in a person. Such people are able to choose the right path from the wrong one on the basis of their instinct. People who possess this line are vibrant and have the tendency of being overly emotional. They can get extremely sensitive about certain issues. An uneven intuition line signifies that the person's intuition may not always be correct.

THE HEALTH LINE

The health line is also referred to as the Hepatica. This line runs diagonally through the palm and starts inside the lifeline near the joint of the palm and the wrist and ends near the beginning of the heart line. It is a little more prominent than the other minor lines.

However, those who do not have this line do not face any health problems. Therefore, we can say that it does not necessarily have a positive or negative effect on the health of an individual.

Ideally, this line should be free of any gaps or marks and the more prominent it is, the better it is said to be. It signifies good health and also indicates that the person has a tendency to recover quickly from an illness. If the line is faint in certain parts, then it means that the person suffers from an illness or general lack of energy and power.

A prominent and well-marked Hepatica also signifies a long life without any major health problems, and denotes physical strength and liveliness.

THE SYMPATHY LINE

This line is situated below the index finger. If this line is straight, then the person is sympathetic and generous. Such people are likely to be social activists and reformists.

THE RASCETTES

They are also called the bracelets and are just below the palm on the wrist. Normally, they are three in number, but in some cases their number may vary.

The first rascette signifies the first twenty-five years of our life, the second rascette indicates middle age and the last one indicates the remaining years of our life.

If the first rascette, which is away from the palm, has gaps it signifies that the person had to struggle in his growing years. Similarly, if the middle or the last rascette shows breaks, then it means in that stage of faced or may face problems life. If a person's middle rascette is the most prominent one, it means that the person has achieved the most in these years of his life both personally and professionally.

Though they do not indicate the longevity of a person's life, if a woman's first rascette curves towards the palm then it indicates that she will either have problems during childbirth, or some gynaecological or urinary problem.

THE FAMILY LINES

These lines are located where the thumb starts from the palm. If they are numerous it means that person will be family-oriented and possessive about his near ones. Similarly, if these lines are less in number, then it signifies that the person is not much emotionally attached to his family.

If this line is thicker towards the side where the index finger is located, then it means that the person was initially emotionally attached to his family. If the line becomes gradually thin on the side where the wrist is located, then it means that the person became less emotionally attached to his family.

A small gap in this line indicates rift with the family and a major break signifies that the person split from his family.

TRAVEL LINES

These lines are located at the side of the palm. Starting from the head line they move forward towards the wrist, ending towards the lunar mount. If these lines are long, then it means that the person will spend more time travelling. If these lines curve upwards, then it symbolizes a fruitful journey. If these lines curve downwards, then it means that the person did not accomplish what he intended to on his journey.

CHILDREN LINES

These lines are located below the little finger in a vertical form. These lines show the possibility of the number of children one may have. But this number can vary depending on one's will to have kids. For example, one may have the possibility of having three children but if a person intends to have only one, they will have one. Therefore, in order to fulfil one's desire, the person will look for ways to have only one child and with the advancement of science, that sure has become easy nowadays.

RELATIONSHIP LINES

These lines are located on the side of the palm between the little finger and the heart line. These lines do not essentially signify marriage. These lines signify those relationships which intense in nature and play a vital role in our lives.

A man may be married but still may not have any relationship lines. It means that the person does not have any personal attachment or bonding in his married life. He may be leading a normal married life without the existence of love and feelings, and his married life may be deficient in intensity.

If there is a prominent relationship line which does not reach the palm, it signifies a strong relationship which came to an end early, but if this line properly reaches the surface of the palm then it signifies a long relationship.

These lines do appear and disappear according to the state of mind of a person while in the relationship and even afterwards. The outcome of a relationship is clearly reflected in these lines. Having more than three relationship lines does not mean that the person has been into as many relationships. It simply states that there was a potential for three or more strong relationships but since the first one persisted, the other ones never came into existence.

RING OF SOLOMON

The ring of Solomon is a small line rising under the finger of Jupiter. It is also a very rare sign and indicates the love for psychic studies and an ability to obtain proficiency in them.

RING OF SATURN

The ring of Saturn is a line which rises between the fingers of Jupiter and Saturn, encircles the finger of Saturn, thus crossing the mount of Saturn completely. This is a mark seldom found. The presence of this mark shows a disposition to jump from one thing to another and not to stick to anything for long enough.

THE GIRDLE OF VENUS

The girdle of Venus is the broken or unbroken kind of semicircle rising between the first and second finger and finishing between the third and fourth.

The presence of this line indicates a highly sensitive and intellectual person with changeable mood and who gets easily offended over little things.

People possessing this mark are capable of rising to the highest level of enthusiasm over anything that engages their fancy, but they rarely remain for long in the same mood—one moment they are in high spirits, in the next moment, they are miserable and despondent.

10

Markings

CROSS

A cross on the Mount of Saturn when touching the line of fate, warns of danger of violence. A cross on the Mount of Venus, when heavily marked, indicates some great trial or fatal influence of affection. A cross by the side of the line of fate, and between it and the lifeline in the plain Mars, denotes opposition in one's career by relatives.

SQUARE

The square is also called the mark of preservation because it shows that the person is protected at that particular point of time from danger. When the line of fate runs through a well-formed square, it denotes one of the greatest crisis in the life of the person, but the square preserves the person from serious loss. When the head line runs through a well-formed square, it is a sign of strength and preservation to the brain. If found on Jupiter, it protects the person from self-ambition. If found on Sun, it protects the person from desire for fame. If found on Mars, it protects the person from enemies.

STAR

Star on Jupiter: A star is a sign of great importance. When a star appears on the Mount of Jupiter, it has distinct meanings, according to its position. When on the highest point of the mount, on the face of the palm, it promises great honour, power and position.

Star on the Mount of Saturn: A star on the Mount of Saturn is not considered auspicious. It indicates some tragedy.

Star on the Mount of Sun: A star on the Mount of Sun brings prosperity; when it is connected with the Sun line, it denotes great fame and name.

Star on the Mount of Mercury: A star in the centre of the Mount of Mercury denotes name, fame and success in science, business, the power of reasoning and also instils good writing skills depending on the type of hand.

11

Health

One of the biggest concerns in a person's life is his health. People are curious to know if there will be any problem in their life regarding their fitness and smooth functioning of the body. The fear of any disability or any untoward incident which may affect their health and the functions of the body is always a matter of concern.

It is not only the state of our physical health but also our emotional state of mind which affects our life greatly. Our state of mind also affects our physical state and vice versa. Therefore, we can say that they are both greatly interrelated. Any sort of strain affects our physical strength and stamina. If there is continuous or prolonged tension in a person's life, it will ultimately sap the energy of a person.

We get to know the state of emotional health by looking at the palm of a person. All the lines, the head line, the fate line, the heart line, etc. tell us something about the state of our mind. Also the number of stress lines on the palm help us to know about the emotional stability or instability in the life of a person. The last line which is to be analysed for determining the health of a person is his lifeline. There should not be any gaps or marks as they indicate problems in the smooth functioning of a person's health. The study and analysis of all these aspects helps us to know the actual state of a person's health.

The shape of the fingers, the hands, the lines—all of these collectively give us knowledge about the person's health. The lesser the number of stress lines, the more balanced and relaxed will be a person's life. Subsequently, people with a short hand and broad fingers tend to be more energetic than people with a long hand and thin fingers. Therefore, what I am trying to point out here is that it is not just one factor which will reflect a person's health.

Other factors that determine our health are worry lines, the size of each mount, and the health line also updates us about the health of a person. Therefore, a careful study of each of these factors point to the physical and emotional stamina of a person.

Lesser number of worry lines, adequate size of the mount, and well-placed and well-marked health line tell us about the physical and emotional well-being of a person.

Therefore, all these reasons and factors can only be known and not changed. It is only the virtues and deeds of a person which can remove or minimize the negativity, if any, on the palm of a person.

LOVE

Love, the most important human emotion, is something which everyone wants to know about. Many young people who come to me have this question on the top of their list: when will they find their true love? Another thing that I find interesting is that not only young people but people of all ages discuss their love life. It's just that with the advancement of age, the priorities in a person's life change. When one is young, love is the foremost thing on a person's mind.

It is believed that people with similar size and shape of lines, hands and fingers have the possibility of a better relationship. They will have similar tastes and dislikes and therefore, there will be better prospects of a successful relationship. But I believe when it comes to love, everything is unexpected. I have observed many people who had almost nothing in common but shared a healthy and loving relationship. The reason for this is that true love can make a person accept and ignore all the flaws a person has, since nobody is perfect.

It is easy to fall in love but much harder to sustain it over the years. It is mutual love, understanding and respect which help a relationship to survive. It is only when either of these go missing, the obstacles in a relationship start surfacing.

The main things to be observed in relationships and love are the heart line, the shape of hand and fingers, and the mount of Venus. Each of these factors enlightens us about the state of relationships in the life of a person. All the sun signs represent a certain element—fire, water, earth or air. It is also the compatibility of each of these elements with the other which plays a major role in the equation between two people.

The mount of Venus tells us the level of emotions and sensitivity in a person. It signifies the passion which is there in a person. Therefore, it also determines the sex life of a person which plays a vital role in love. It is the level of desire and energy that is present in a person which affects and keeps the relationship alive. For a vivacious relationship, the mount of Venus should be full in size in both the partners. It indicates that the level of love, desire, care and understanding is the same in both which fulfils the expectation from their relationship. Similarly, if the size of the mount of Venus is small in both, then it means that they lack desire and the need to keep the relationship vibrant. They are satisfied with the company of each other and it is togetherness that they share which is providing them with contentment.

Likewise, if the shape of the thumbs of both the people is the same and ideal in nature, then it signifies that both have a tendency to value their relationship more than their ego and their temper. They will have a tendency to bend their egos and beliefs for the happiness of their partner and contentment in the relationship.

The heart line also helps us know about the emotional state of a person. This line determines the warmth in a person regarding his personal relationships. If there are no breaks in the heart line, it signifies that the person will have a sensitive nature, and will therefore be caring in relationships. Also people who have a curved heart line are more warm and expressive in love, whereas people whose heart line is flat do not show and discuss their feelings easily. It is also ideal for the heart line to end at almost the same place as their partner.

When the heart lines end at different places or the sizes of the Mount of Venus vary, there are chances of conflict between the couple. However, any conflict can be overcome by love and understanding.

HAPPINESS

Another aspect that people ask me very frequently about is happiness and satisfaction in life. It generally indicates that the person is overly concerned or is presently facing some problem.

Happiness has a lot to do with contentment and subsequently all the aspects of a person's life. If one aspect of a person's life is creating a problem, it will result in unhappiness, no matter how well the other things are going. It is very rare for every area of our life to be as we expect them. Therefore, it is very important to be content and satisfied with what we already have instead of what we do not have. We should count our blessings.

Therefore, happiness is always around but instead of looking for happiness we look for various reasons to be unhappy. So, instead, I suggest people make efforts or at least count the various reasons for their happiness. Problems are part and parcel of life and without them there will be no personal growth and appreciation of what we possess. Happiness depends on the outlook and approach of a person towards life.

First, it is the lifeline of a person which helps us know the state of a person's mind. It signifies the energy and stamina of a person along with the direction of his/her life. If a person is well aware of his goals and ambitions, he will have the urge to achieve them. Hence, he will be making efforts and working towards achieving it. This direction of a person's life occupies his mind and gives him a purpose in life.

Also, the shape of a person's hand determines the quality of a person's life. People with broad hands are more likely to be successful in life and therefore their sense of achievement will instil happiness in their life. It is not just one factor which helps us know the element of happiness.

What one should observe next is the head line of a person. It informs us about the mental ability, intelligence and confidence in a person. This line informs us if the person is fully utilizing the intelligence that he was born with. Inadequate utilization means that the person is not making full efforts and therefore, he will not be rewarded for his efforts as much as he deserves. This is due to the reason that the person lacks the direction in which he should channelize his intelligence.

The lesser the number of lines on the hand, the happier the person will be. More lines on the hand indicate more stress, worry and anxiety. Lesser lines also indicate a higher level of confidence and faith in one's own ability. The more confident a person, the happier and self-assured he will be.

People usually discuss or ask about that area of their life which has not been satisfactory. Therefore, finding the reason, cause or remedy to rectify that problem means that eventually eradication of that problem will result in happiness.